Management of the Hospitalized Patient with Diabetes

Editor

CELIA ANN LEVESQUE

CRITICAL CARE NURSING CLINICS OF NORTH AMERICA

www.ccnursing.theclinics.com

March 2025 • Volume 37 • Number 1

ELSEVIER

1600 John F. Kennedy Boulevard • Suite 1800 • Philadelphia, Pennsylvania, 19103-2899

http://www.theclinics.com

CRITICAL CARE NURSING CLINICS OF NORTH AMERICA Volume 37, Number 1
March 2025 ISSN 0899-5885, ISBN-13: 978-0-443-29604-8

Editor: Kerry Holland
Developmental Editor: Sukirti Singh

Critical Care Nursing Clinics of North America (ISSN 0899-5885) is published quarterly by Elsevier Inc., 360 Park Avenue South, New York, NY 10010-1710. Months of issue are March, June, September, and December. Business and Editorial Offices: 1600 John F. Kennedy Blvd., Suite 1800, Philadelphia, PA 19103-2899. Periodicals postage paid at New York, NY and additional mailing offices. Subscription prices are $166.00 per year for US individuals, $100.00 per year for US students and residents, $206.00 per year for Canadian individuals, $230.00 per year for international individuals, $115.00 per year for international students/residents and $100.00 per year for Canadian students/residents. For institutional access pricing please contact Customer Service via the contact information below. To receive student/resident rate, orders must be accompanied by name of affiliated institution, data of term, and the *signature* of program/residency co-ordinator on institution letterhead. Orders will be billed at individual rate until proof of status is received. Foreign air speed delivery is included in all *Clinics* subscription prices. All prices are subject to change without notice. Orders, claims, and journal inquiries: Please visit our Support Hub page https://service.elsevier.com for assistance.

Reprints. For copies of 100 or more of articles in this publication, please contact the Commercial Reprints Department, Elsevier Inc., 360 Park Avenue South, New York, New York, 10010-1710; Tel.: 212-633-3874, Fax: 212-633-3820, and E-mail: reprints@elsevier.com.

Critical Care Nursing Clinics of North America is covered in *MEDLINE/PubMed (Index Medicus), International Nursing Index, Nursing Citation Index, Cumulative Index to Nursing and Allied Health Literature, and RNdex Top 100.*

Contributors

EDITOR

CELIA ANN LEVESQUE, APRN, NP-C, CNS-BC, CDCES, BC-ADM
Advanced Practice Registered Nurse, Department of Endocrine Neoplasia and Hormonal Disorders, The University of Texas MD Anderson Cancer Center, Houston, Texas, USA

AUTHORS

VERONICA BRADY, PhD, MSN, BSN
Assistant Professor, Department of Research, Cizik School of Nursing at UTHealth Houston, Nurse Practitioner, The University of Texas MD Anderson Cancer Center, Houston, Texas, USA

ANNE BRINKMAN, DNP, APRN, AGNP-C
Advanced Practice Registered Nurse, Department of Endocrine Neoplasia and Hormonal Disorders, The University of Texas MD Anderson Cancer Center, Houston, Texas, USA

KATE CRAWFORD, RN, MSN, ANP-C
Nurse Practitioner, Velocity Clinical Research, Dallas, Texas, USA

HSIAO-HUI JU, DNP, APRN, FNP-BC, CNE
Assistant Professor, Department of Undergraduate Studies, Cizik School of Nursing at UTHealth Houston, Houston, Texas, USA

CELIA ANN LEVESQUE, APRN, NP-C, CNS-BC, CDCES, BC-ADM
Advanced Practice Registered Nurse, Department of Endocrine Neoplasia and Hormonal Disorders, The University of Texas MD Anderson Cancer Center, Houston, Texas, USA

ELAINE MADUZIA, MSN, MHA, RN, CPHQ
Diabetes Care and Education Specialist, Nurse Navigator Diabetes, Quality Department, Houston Methodist, The Woodlands Hospital, The Woodlands, Texas, USA

DEBORAH L. McCREA, EdD, MSN, RN, FNP-BC, CNS, CNE, CEN, CFRN, EMT-P
Assistant Professor of Clinical Nursing, Department of Graduate Studies, Cizik School of Nursing at UTHealth Houston, Houston, Texas, USA

MARJORIE R. ORTIZ, MSN, RN, AGPCNP-BC, BC-ADM
Advanced Practice Provider, Department of Endocrine Neoplasia and Hormonal Disorders, The University of Texas MD Anderson Cancer Center, Houston, Texas, USA

DENISE ANN PALMA, MS, MBA, MHA, RD, LD, CDCES, BC-ADM
Diabetes Educator Coordinator, Department of Endocrine Neoplasia and Hormonal Disorders, The University of Texas MD Anderson Cancer Center, Houston, Texas, USA

KATHLEEN J. PINCUS, PharmD, BCPS, BCACP, CDCES
Associate Professor, Department of Practice, Sciences, and Health Outcomes Research, University of Maryland School of Pharmacy, Baltimore, Maryland, USA

CHARMAINE D. ROCHESTER-EYEGUOKAN, PharmD, BCACP, CDCES
Professor, Department of Practice, Sciences, and Health Outcomes Research, University of Maryland School of Pharmacy, Baltimore, Maryland, USA

VERONICA SANCHEZ, BSN, RN, SCRN
Staff RN, Intensive Care Unit, Houston Methodist, The Woodlands Hospital, The Woodlands, Texas, USA

MILI VAKHARIA, MSN, APRN, FNP-C, CDCES
Assistant Professor, Division of Pediatric Diabetes and Endocrinology, Department of Pediatrics, Baylor College of Medicine, Texas Children's Hospital, Houston, Texas, USA

TINA WYNN, RD, LD, CDCES
Certified Diabetes Care and Education Specialist, Department of Endocrine Neoplasia and Hormonal Disorders, The University of Texas MD Anderson Cancer Center, Houston, Texas, USA

Contents

> Hyperglycemia and diabetes place hospitalized patients at a greater risk for serious complications such as infections, diabetic ketoacidosis, hyperosmolar hyperglycemic state, dehydration, electrolyte imbalances, polypharmacy, and lengthened hospitalization. Identification and proper treatment of hyperglycemia and diabetes are essential to reduce morbidity and mortality, as well as to conserve limited health care resources. This article will summarize the current American Diabetes Association and Endocrine Society recommendations for the management of hospitalized patients with hyperglycemia and diabetes. It will discuss the diagnostic criteria for the identification of diabetes and hyperglycemia, glycemic targets, pharmacologic management of hyperglycemia, and the transition to outpatient care.

> Many hospitals have a lack of Certified Diabetes Care and Education Specialists leaving a gap in providing the education necessary for patients with diabetes to manage their diabetes after discharge. Training hospital nurses to become diabetes nurse champions can help fill in the gap. In addition to providing the patient with diabetes education, the diabetes nurse champion can advocate for glycemic management in the hospital to improve glycemic goals, reducing the incidence of hypoglycemia and severe hyperglycemia. This article will discuss ways to train nurses to be diabetes nurse champions.

> The prevalence of pediatric diabetes continues to rise in the United States and worldwide. There are various forms of pediatric diabetes including type 1, type 2, and maturity onset diabetes of youth. The treatment depends on each unique type of diabetes and must be taken into consideration for patients based on presentation and clinical setting. There is limited literature supporting the use of noninsulin medications to manage pediatric diabetes in an inpatient setting. This article focuses on noninsulin medication management of children and adolescents presenting with hyperglycemia in acute care settings, both critically and noncritically ill.

Perioperative evaluation and management of diabetes mellitus is vital to minimize adverse complications before, during, and after surgery. It requires a multidisciplinary approach including the surgery team, anesthesia, endocrinology or internal medicine, and other specialties as needed. This article will discuss the effects of surgery and anesthesia on blood glucose, preoperative evaluation of the person with diabetes, glycemic targets for surgery, adjustment of diabetes medications the day before surgery, in the preoperative, intraoperative, and postoperative areas, management of blood glucose in the preoperative, intraoperative, and postoperative periods, and management of hypoglycemia.

Diabetes self-management education and support (DSME/S) creates the pillars necessary for a person with diabetes (PWD) to build self-confidence in how to manage a diagnosis of diabetes. Health care organizations should remain flexible and adaptable to seeking new methods in providing patient education particularly a PWD. As diabetes diagnosis continues to grow along with different diabetes tools and technology, health care organizations should consider embracing change by implementing the use DSME/S, developing a diabetes management inpatient team, and acquiring Certified Diabetes Care and Education Specialists.

Diabetic ketoacidosis (DKA) and euglycemic DKA are both diabetes-related emergencies. Individuals with DKA can experience extremely elevated hyperglycemia exceeding 250 mg/dL. Although DKA is more frequently observed in people with type 1 diabetes (T1DM), euglycemic DKA, which is characterized by mildly elevated or nearly normal blood glucose at levels below 200 mg/dL, has recently been linked to the use of SGLT-2 inhibitors generally used for type 2 diabetes mellitus (T2DM). Without the substantial hyperglycemia associated with DKA, euglycemic DKA may be clinically overlooked. The pathophysiology, precipitating factors, clinical presentations, treatments, and evaluations of euglycemic DKA and DKA are reviewed.

CRITICAL CARE NURSING CLINICS OF NORTH AMERICA

SERIES OF RELATED INTEREST

Nursing Clinics of North America http://www.nursing.theclinics.com
Critical Care Clinics www.criticalcare.theclinics.com

THE CLINICS ARE AVAILABLE ONLINE!
Access your subscription at:
www.theclinics.com

Preface

Management of Diabetes in the Hospitalized Patient

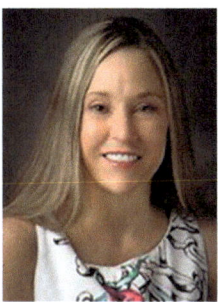

Celia Ann Levesque, APRN, NP-C, CNS-BC, CDCES, BC-ADM
Editor

According to the National Diabetes Statistics report published May 15, 2024 from the Centers for Disease Control and Prevention, 38.4 million Americans (11.6%) have diabetes. Approximately one in six hospitalized patients have diabetes. Inpatient hyperglycemia and hypoglycemia are associated with increased morbidity, mortality, length of stay, rehospitalization, and cost of care. Hospitalized patients with diabetes are at increased risk for infection, poor wound healing, electrolyte imbalances, dehydration, malnutrition, ketoacidosis, and hyperosmolar hyperglycemic state. Inpatient diabetes management programs based on published guidelines improve blood glucose and reduce the risk for diabetes-related adverse outcomes. Management of common issues in hospitalized patients with diabetes is included in this *issue of Critical Care Nursing Clinics of North America.*

- "Management of the Hospitalized Patients with Hyperglycemia" discusses glycemic targets for hospitalized patients, recommended treatment of hyperglycemia based on published standards of care, and transition to outpatient care.
- "Training Hospital Nurses to be Diabetes Champions" discusses the common issue that most hospitals do not employ enough Diabetes Care and Education Specialists to meet patient needs, so training nurses to be diabetes champions provides greatly needed diabetes survival skills training for patients to be discharged home safely.
- "Non–Insulin Diabetes Medications in Hospitalized Children and Adolescents" covers the approved diabetes medications for children and adolescents and how they are used in the hospital setting.
- "Using Diabetes Technology in Hospitalized Patients" discusses the use of continuous glucose monitors and insulin pumps in the hospitalized patient.

Crit Care Nurs Clin N Am 37 (2025) xi–xii
https://doi.org/10.1016/j.cnc.2024.11.001
0899-5885/25/© 2024 Published by Elsevier Inc.

ccnursing.theclinics.com

- "Managing Heart Disease in Persons with Diabetes" discusses the risk factors for the development of heart disease in patients with diabetes and current standards of care by professional organizations.
- "Diabetes Management in the Critical Care Setting: Insulin Infusions" discusses the use of insulin drips in the critical care setting and how to transition from intravenous to subcutaneous insulin therapy.
- "Current Medical Nutrition Therapy Recommendations for the Person with Diabetes" discusses general nutrition recommendations for people with diabetes and the risk for malnutrition after hospitalization, how to screen for malnutrition, and various ways to treat malnutrition, including supplements and enteral and parenteral nutrition.
- "Management of Hypertension in Patients with Diabetes" discusses target blood pressure in people with diabetes and current treatment recommendations, including lifestyle modification and medication.
- "Management of Immunotherapy-induced Type 1 Diabetes" discusses the immunotherapy medications that are associated with the development of type 1 diabetes, the comparison of immunotherapy-induced type 1 diabetes and autoimmune type 1 diabetes, monitoring for diabetes-related ketoacidosis, and treatment recommendations.
- "Hypoglycemia in Hospitalized Patients with Diabetes" discusses the risk factors for development of hypoglycemia, and the treatment and prevention of hypoglycemia in hospitalized patients with diabetes.
- "Current Recommendations for Insulin Therapy in the Hospitalized Patient" discusses the various insulins on the US market and common insulin regimens used in hospitalized patients.
- "Perioperative Management of the Patient with Diabetes Mellitus" discusses the current recommendations for management of blood glucose before, during, and after surgery.
- "Diabetes Education for the Hospitalized Patient" discusses a team approach in providing diabetes survival skills based on the Association of Diabetes Care and Education Specialists ADCES7 Self-Care Behaviors to help the patient with transitioning to self-care at home after discharge.
- "Euglycemic Diabetic Ketoacidosis: How Is It Different from Diabetic Ketoacidosis" compares diabetic ketoacidosis and euglycemic diabetic ketoacidosis, including the pathogenesis, risk factors, signs and symptoms, and treatment.

DISCLOSURES

The author does not have any disclosures, nor commercial or financial conflicts of interest and has not received any funding sources.

Celia Ann Levesque, APRN, NP-C, CNS-BC, CDCES, BC-ADM
Department of Endocrine Neoplasia and
Hormonal Disorders
The University of Texas MD Anderson Cancer Center
1515 Holcomb Boulevard
Houston, TX 77030, USA

E-mail address:
clevesqu@mdanderson.org

Management of the Hospitalized Patient with Hyperglycemia

Kate Crawford, RN, MSN, ANP-C

KEYWORDS

- Diabetes • Hyperglycemia • Hypoglycemia • Insulin • Hospitalized patients

KEY POINTS

- Diabetes and hyperglycemia in hospitalized patients increase the risk for serious complications such as worsened infections, prolonged hospitalization, polypharmacy, DKA, and HHS.
- Identifying and treating hyperglycemia and diabetes in hospitalized patients are associated with reduced morbidity and mortality.
- The goal of inpatient hyperglycemia treatment is to achieve glycemic targets while minimizing hypoglycemia.

INTRODUCTION

Diabetes is one of the most common chronic illnesses in the United States. The Center for Diesease Control (CDC) reports approximately 38 million people or 11.6% of the US population have diabetes, increased from 8.3% of the population in 2011.[1] Of those patients, more than 8 million are undiagnosed. Thirty-eight percent of adults have prediabetes with nearly 50% of those over 65 having prediabetes.[1]

It is, therefore, reasonable to assume the proportion of hospitalized patien with overt diabetes or hyperglycemia to be significant. It is estimated that patients with diabetes account for more than 25% of noncritically ill hospitalized patients[2] and 12% to 25% of patients without a diagnosis of diabetes are expected to become hyperglycemic while admitted.[3] Diabetes was listed as the fifth most common diagnosis in hospitalized patients in 2018.[4]

Hyperglycemia and diabetes place hospitalized patients at greater risk for serious complications such as infections, diabetic ketoacidosis (DKA), hyperosmolar hyperglycemic state (HHS), dehydration, electrolyte imbalances, polypharmacy, lengthened hospitalization and increased morbidity, and increased rates of readmission.[5] It is, therefore, essential that health care professionals be able to identify and manage this common condition to prevent serious complications.

Velocity Clinical Research, 7777 Forest Lane C685, Dallas, TX 75230, USA
E-mail address: kcrawford@velocityclinical.com

Crit Care Nurs Clin N Am 37 (2025) 1–10
https://doi.org/10.1016/j.cnc.2024.08.005
0899-5885/25/© 2024 Elsevier Inc. All rights reserved, including those for text and data mining, AI training, and similar technologies.

This article will discuss the identification and assessment of hyperglycemia in hospitalized patients, glycemic targets, treatments, and transition to outpatient care. The American Diabetes Association (ADA) 2024 Standards of Care[6] and the Endocrine Society's Clinical Practice Guideline for the Management of Hyperglycemia in Hospitalized Adult Patients in Noncritical Care settings[7] will serve as the main references for this article.

IDENTIFICATION AND ASSESSMENT OF DIABETES AND HYPERGLYCEMIA

While diabetes was the fifth most common diagnosis in hospitalized patients in 2018,[4] hyperglycemia and diabetes can be viewed as less important than other more urgent admission diagnoses such as myocardial infarction, delaying identification, and treatment of hyperglycemia. As hyperglycemia is well known to contribute to worse outcomes for hospitalized patients,[5] the prompt identification and treatment of hyperglycemia and diabetes are, therefore, critical to prevent serious complications.

IDENTIFICATION OF HYPERGLYCEMIA

Hyperglycemia in hospitalized patients is defined as glucose values greater than or equal to 140 mg/dL. A1c Values greater than or equal to 6.5 on admission indicate diabetes.

A1c should be obtained for all pts with a previous diagnosis of diabetes or in any patient with hyperglycemia (glucose $\geq$140 mg/dL) upon admission if A1C value within past 3 months is not available.[6]

GLYCEMIC GOALS
Critically Ill

The Normoglycemia in Intensive Care Evaluation and Survival Using Glucose Algorithm Regulation (NICE-SUGAR) trial[8] resulted in a re-evaluation of glycemic goals in critically ill patients. Patients in the intensive treatment arm (glucose values 80–110 mg/dL) did not derive a significant treatment benefit but did experience 10 to 15 times increased rates of hypoglycemia as well as slightly higher, but significant increase in mortality. The ADA and Endocrine Society[6,7] therefore recommend glucose values between 140 and 180 mg/dL for most critically ill individuals with hyperglycemia on insulin treatment.

Noncritically Ill

There are not yet widely accepted glycemic targets for noncritically ill hospitalized pts.[6] Glucose values between 100 and 180 mg/dL are suggested, regardless of prior history of diabetes.[6]

Unnumbered Box 1. Evaluation of glucose levels in hospitalized patients		
	Critically ill	Noncritically ill
Glucose	140–180	100–180

Glycemic targets should always be individualized to each patient. Less aggressive goals (glucose >250 mg/dL) may be appropriate for patients at high risk for hypoglycemia such as the elderly, patients with renal or hepatic dysfunction, patients with altered mental status, or in those patients who would not benefit from tight glycemic control such as the terminally ill or patients in palliative care.[6,7]

Patients with a history of diabetes should have the diagnosis clearly documented in the medical record with a description of the outpatient medication regimen, level of glycemic control (if known), and frequency of hypoglycemia.[6,7]

Interpretation of A1c and Glucose Values			
	Diabetes	IGT	Normoglycemia
A1c	>6.5	5.7–6.4	≤5.6
Fasting glucose	>126	100–125	<100

A1c should be interpreted with caution in pts with certain disorders as it may not be indicative of their usual glycemic control,[6,7] see **Table 1**.

GLUCOSE MONITORING
Point of Care

The ADA[6] recommends point-of-care (POC) glucose monitoring for all patients previously diagnosed with diabetes and for those patients with glucose values greater than 140 mg/dL on admission. Glucose monitoring should be considered in patients at high risk for developing hyperglycemia while admitted to detect any elevations in glucose[6] (**Table 2**).

FREQUENCY OF MONITORING

The frequency of glucose monitoring depends on the PO status of the patient.

Unnumbered Box 2. Monitoring Glucose Levels		
Meals/bolus feeds	NPO/Continuous enteral/parenteral nutrition	Insulin drip
AC and HS	Q 4–6 h	Per protocol

For patients who are eating or receiving bolus enteral feeding, glucose should be checked before the actual meal or bolus feed, not at prespecified times. This can pose challenges in hospitals that offer on demand meals, but it is important the caregiver and patient work together to ensure glucose is checked at the appropriate time.

In patients who are NPO, or receiving continuous enteral or parenteral nutrition, glucose should be checked at minimum every 6 hours.

Pts receiving intravenous (IV) insulin should have glucose monitored as specified per the drip protocol.

CONTINUOUS GLUCOSE MONITORING

The ADA and Endocrine Society[6,7] both support the use of continuous glucose monitoring (CGM) for hospitalized pts with types 1 and 2 diabetes previously prescribed the devices, especially for insulin-treated pts at high risk for hypoglycemia[6] (see **Table 5**).

Table 1 Conditions that interfere with A1c interpretation	
Anemia	Hemoglobinopathies
Chronic renal failure	Alcoholism or drug use
Significant glycemic variability	Pts receiving blood products
Nutritional deficits	Recent significant blood loss

Table 2
Patients at high risk for developing hyperglycemia

Overweight or Obesity BMI >30	Age >45
Hypertension	Hyperlipidemia
Steroid use	Enteral/parenteral nutrition
Surgical patients	Pancreatic patients
Octreotide use	\Immunosuppressants

CGM is particularly useful for patients who experience nocturnal hypoglycemia and for patients with diminished hypoglycemia awareness. CGM values should be verified with POC testing for all insulin dosing and assessment of hypoglycemia.[6,7]

CGM must be removed prior to any X-ray, mammography, DEXA scan, fluoroscopy, CT, or MRI. CGM data may not be accurate in certain patient populations[6] (**Table 3**). In these instances, POC testing should be implemented.

TREATMENT OF DIABETES AND HYPERGLYCEMIA

Patients who were previously prescribed with insulin should continue their usual regimen with appropriate modifications as needed for alterations in PO intake, renal function, etc.[6,7] Treatment with insulin and/or other therapies should be initiated for glucose values persistently greater than or equal to 180 mg/dL.[6] Insulin is the usual recommended treatment for inpatient hyperglycemia due to efficacy and flexibility.[6,7]

The schedule and route of insulin administration depend on the acuity of care; critically ill versus noncritically ill.

Critically Ill

Continuous IV infusions of insulin using standardized protocols are the recommended treatment of hyperglycemia in critically ill patients.[6,7] There are numerous validated insulin protocols that are beyond the scope of this article.

Noncritically Ill

In the noncritically ill patient, scheduled insulin programs are recommended which include basal, bolus, and correctional insulin.[6,7] The type of insulin regimen will depend upon the PO status of the patient.

Unnumbered Table 2. Recommended Insulin regimens and glucose monitoring based on PO intake.

	NPO	Continuous enteral/ parenteral feeds	PO/Bolus feed
Monitor	Q6	Q6	AC & HS
Insulin	Basal + correction	Basal + correction	basal + bolus + correction

Table 3
Conditions/Medications that interfere with continuous glucose monitoring accuracy

Patients with Extensive Skin Infections	Hypoperfusion or Hypovolemia
Vasoactive or pressor therapy	Acetaminophen > 4 g/d
Dopamine	Vitamin C >500 mg/d
Hydroxyurea	

Basal Insulins

Basal insulin is utilized to control elevations from hepatic glucose output between meals and overnight. Basal insulin is usually administered once daily but can be administered twice a day for intermediate acting insulin such as NPH or if more flexibility and opportunity for adjustment is required. Basal insulin is given without regard to PO intake. It is critical to remember that patients with type 1 diabetes are absolutely insulin deficient and require basal insulin regardless of PO intake. Basal insulin should never be withheld from pts with type 1 diabetes.

The available basal insulins in the United States are as follows.

- Intermediate acting: NPH
- Long acting: Detemir, Degludec, Glargine, Glargine biosimilar.

Prandial or Bolus Insulin

Bolus insulin is administered to control glycemic elevations that result from PO intake. Insulins used are rapid or short-acting and should be administered with meals. It is important to administer bolus insulin when the patient is actually eating as inappropriate timing of bolus insulin without regard to meals can result in hypoglycemia. Carbohydrate counting, administering a certain amount of prandial insulin depending on the carbohydrate content of the meal, is not recommended for hospitalized patients with type 2 diabetes; however, patients with type 1 diabetes may continue utilizing insulin to carb ratios for prandial dosing if the facility is capable of supporting its use.[7] Rapid or short acting insulins available in the United States are as follows.

- Short acting: Regular insulin
- Rapid acting: Aspart, Glulisine, Lispro (several forms)

Correctional Insulin

Correctional insulin is an additional dose of short or rapid acting insulin administered with a bolus dose to correct for hyperglycemia prior to a meal or insulin administered every 6 hours in patients who are NPO. Correctional insulin can be used alone in specific situations or in combination with scheduled insulin therapy.

Premixed Insulins

Premixed insulins contain a fixed percentage of basal and bolus insulins premixed in the solution such as 50/50, 75/25, and 70/30. They are administered twice a day, prior to breakfast and dinner. While these preparations have been shown to have similar efficacy in glycemic control, they also increase the risk for hypoglycemia and are not recommended for hospitalized patients.[6] Basal bolus regimens are preferred.[6,7]

In patients who are NPO, scheduled basal insulin (one or twice a day) or basal plus correction insulin (Q 4–6 hours) is recommended.

In pts who are eating, intermediate-acting or long-acting basal insulin (once or twice a day) with prandial administration of a rapid-acting or short-acting insulin prior to meals plus correctional insulin is recommended.

In pts without a history of diabetes and glucose values 140 to 180 mg/dL, the limited use correctional insulin alone is acceptable. However, it is recommended that patients receiving correctional insulin with 2 glucose values greater than 180 within 24 hours be prescribed scheduled insulin therapy (basal or basal bolus) regardless of diabetes history prior to admission.[7]

It must be emphasized that the patients with type 1 diabetes are absolutely insulin deficient and must have basal insulin to prevent DKA, regardless of PO intake. It is never appropriate to withhold insulin in patients with type 1 diabetes.

Insulin Pumps and Automated Insulin Delivery Systems

In patients who were previously utilizing insulin pumps or automated insulin delivery systems (AIDS), the ADA and Endocrine Society recommend continuing these devices if the patient is capable of safely utilizing the device and access to providers' proficient with their use are available.[6,7] If the staff is not proficient with this technology and the hospitalization is expected to be longer than 1 to 2 days, it is recommended the device be discontinued and the patient transitioned to a scheduled insulin regimen.[7] Insulin pumps and AIDs are not appropriate for use in certain populations and should be discontinued for:

- Impaired level of consciousness
- Inability to appropriately adjust pump settings
- Critical illness
- DKA or HHS

Noninsulin Therapies

As previously stated, insulin is the preferred treatment for hyperglycemia in hospitalized patients; however, some oral medications may be utilized in appropriate circumstances.

Dipeptidyl Peptidase-4 Inhibitors

In pts with type 2 diabetes and mild hyperglycemia, (A1c < 7.5% and glucose < 180 mg/dL), both the ADA and Endocrine Society[6,7] endorse the use of either dipeptidyl peptidase-4 (DPPiv) inhibitors (sitagliptin, saxagliptin, linagliptin, and alogliptin) plus correctional insulin, or scheduled insulin therapy. In patients prescribed with insulin prior to admission, this recommendation only applies to those patients receiving less than 0.6 units of insulin per kilogram per day. If glycemia is persistently greater than 180 mg/dL on DPPiv + correctional insulin, basal/bolus treatment should be initiated.

Sodium-Glucose Transporter 2

It is recommended that patients with diabetes and heart failure continue sodium-glucose transporter 2 (SGLT2) medications (bexagliflozin, canagliflozin, dapagliflozin, empagliflozin, and ertugliflozin) as these medications have indications for improved heart failure outcomes.[6]

Incretin Therapies

Incretin-based injectable therapies such as Semaglutide, Tirzepatide, and Dulaglutide should be discontinued in hospitalized patients as they alter GI mobility and delay gastric emptying. For anticipated admissions, incretins should be held at least 1 week prior to admission.

See **Table 4** for other noninsulin diabetes medications and their indications for use in hospitalized patients.

SPECIAL CIRCUMSTANCES
Steroids

Glucocorticoid use is common in hospitalized patients and can cause hyperglycemia in 50% to 86% of patients receiving supraphysiologic doses, regardless of previous

Table 4
Noninsulin Diabetes Medications and Indications for use in Hospitalized Patients

Medications	Use in Hospital

Sulfonylureas:
  Glimepiride, Glipizide, Glyburide
	Discontinue: high risk for hypoglycemia in
	  unpredictable PO intake, fasting, renal insufficiency

Meglitinides:
  Nateglinide, Repaglinide
	Discontinue: high risk for hypoglycemia in
	  unpredictable PO intake, fasting, renal insufficiency

Thiazolidinediones:
  Pioglitazone
	Minimal risk for hypoglycemia. May continue in stable
	  patients. *Do not initiate in pts at risk for edema, CHF*

Biguanides:
  Metformin
	Hold for renal insufficiency: creatinine: 1.4 women, 1.5
	  men, contrast studies. *Do not initiate in pts with
	  nausea, vomiting, or diarrhea*

Alpha glucosidase inhibitors:
  Acarbose, Miglitol
	Discontinue: high risk for hypoglycemia in
	  unpredictable PO intake, fasting, renal insufficiency
	  Do not initiate in pts with nausea, vomiting, or diarrhea

diabetes diagnosis.[9] There is no consensus on the treatment for glucocorticoid hyperglycemia. The Endocrine Society recommends either intermittent doses of NPH insulin Q 4 to 6 hours with each dose of intermediate-acting steroid or basal bolus regimens for longer acting steroids.[7] Steroid use typically disproportionately affects postprandial glucose values. Patients previously prescribed basal bolus regimens receiving steroids may require significant dosage increases of 40% to 60% of their usual prandial doses.[6]

PARENTERAL/ENTERAL NUTRITION
Enteral Feeding

Patients receiving enteral nutrition who were previously prescribed basal insulin should continue to receive basal insulin. The nutritional component of continuous enteral feeding can be covered with Q 6 hour scheduled doses of prandial insulin plus additional correctional insulin for hyperglycemia.[6]

Alternately, NPH insulin can also be used Q 8 to 12 hours.[6] In patients receiving nocturnal enteral feeding, NPH insulin may also be used to cover the shorter duration of feeding time. If continuous enteral feeding is interrupted in patients receiving insulin therapy, IV dextrose should be administered and the patient should be monitored closely for hypoglycemia.[6]

Patients receiving bolus enteral feeding should receive prandial insulin plus correctional insulin as needed for hyperglycemia prior to each bolus feed.

Parenteral Nutrition

Patient receiving parenteral nutrition should also continue basal insulin if previously prescribed, however, the nutritional insulin component can be added directly to the IV solution. The patient should also have Q 6-hour correctional insulin for hyperglycemia as needed. If the patient requires frequent subcutaneous insulin correction, the amount of insulin added to the parenteral solution should be increased.[6]

As insulin is added to the solution in parenteral nutrition, there is less risk for hypoglycemia if the infusion is interrupted.

HYPOGLYCEMIA

Avoidance of hypoglycemia should be the primary safety concern when treating hospitalized patients with hyperglycemia.

Hypoglycemia is classified based on glucose value and the severity of symptoms.

Unnumbered Box 3. Monitoring Glucose Levels for the severity of symptoms	
	Glucose
Level 1	<70
Level 2	<54
Level 3	Severe event with altered mental status and/or requires assistance for treatment

Hospitalized patients are at increased risk for hypoglycemia due to unpredictable PO intake, changes in medications, interruption of enteral feeding, and inappropriate timing of insulin in addition to the risks outlined in **Table 5**.

Standardized nurse-initiated hypoglycemia protocols for glucose less than 70 mg/dL should be in place for all patients at risk for hypoglycemia.

Treatment of hypoglycemia is dependent on the patients' mental state, PO status, and degree of hypoglycemia.

For patients who are NPO, or unable to swallow, treat with 12 to 25 g of IV dextrose 50%.

For patients who are able to swallow: 15 g of oral glucose is preferred.

Glucose should be rechecked 15 minutes after treatment and steps repeated if glucose is not greater than 70 mg/dL.

Glucagon IM/SQ or intranasal can be utilized in patients who are unable to swallow and do not have IV access.

All episodes of hypoglycemia should be investigated for contributing factors such as change in PO status, stopped or interrupted IV dextrose or enteral feeding, or inappropriate insulin timing so additional episodes can be prevented.

Transition to Outpatient Care

The readmission rate for patients with diabetes is double that for patient without diabetes.[6] It is, therefore, critically important that patients are adequately prepared for the transition to outpatient care to prevent readmission in this high-risk population. The transition from inpatient care to home can be overwhelming for patients and caregivers. There are often numerous new medications and skills that must be mastered in a short amount of time. Discharge planning should, therefore, begin as soon as possible to facilitate a smooth transition and allow for adequate learning time.

Patients with diabetes and hyperglycemia should receive, at minimum, education in the following areas prior to discharge.[6,7]

- When and how to administer all medications
- Prescriptions for new and chronic medications

Table 5 Patients at high risk for hypoglycemia	
>65 years Old	BMI < 27
Total daily dose of insulin $\geq$ 0.6 u/kg	Type 1 diabetes
Renal insufficiency: CKD or eGFR <60	Altered mental status
Malignancy	Pancreatic disease
Recent hypoglycemia	Hypoglycemia unawareness

- When and how to perform BG monitoring
- Individualized glucose goals
- Basic medical nutritional counseling
- Signs, symptoms, and treatment of hypoglycemia
- Signs, symptoms, and treatment of hyperglycemia
- Emergency contacts following hospital discharge
- Follow-up appointments
- Sick day management
- Sharps disposal instructions and supplies

Providers must ensure that patients and caregivers have adequate resources and knowledge to manage their diabetes prior to discharge. If available, a certified diabetes educator can be an excellent resource for patients, caregivers, and staff to provide diabetes education and skills training.

Summary

While the data are limited supporting a unified approach to inpatient hyperglycemic management, the American Diabetes Association 2024 Standards of Care and the Endocrine Society's Clinical Practice Guideline for the Management of Hyperglycemia in Hospitalized Adult Patients in Noncritical Care Settings offer guidance. Patients with diabetes and hyperglycemia should have thorough assessments and monitoring for hyperglycemia. Treatment of hyperglycemia should be administered in a physiologic, scheduled regimen which includes basal/bolus/correctional components that minimize the risk for hypoglycemia. Patients should be adequately be prepared for discharge and the transition to home care to improve outcomes and minimize readmissions.

CLINICS CARE POINTS

- Hyperglycemia, no matter the cause, requires treatment to prevent serious complications.
- Never withhold basal insulin from patients with type 1 diabetes.
- Insulin should be administered in scheduled, physiologic fashion.
- Patients receiving correctional insulin with 2 glucose values greater than 180 within 24 hours should be prescribed scheduled insulin therapy.

DISCLOSURE

The author has no disclosures.

REFERENCES

1. Centers for Disease Control and Prevention. National Diabetes Statistics Report. 2024. Available at: https://www.cdc.gov/diabetes/php/data-research/index.html. Accessed May 15, 2024.
2. Kufeldt J, Kovarova M, Adolph M, et al. Prevalence and distribution of diabetes mellitus in a maximum care hospital: urgent need for HbA1c-screening. Exp Clin Endocrinol Diabetes 2018;126(2):123–9.
3. Cook CB, Kongable GL, Potter DJ, et al. Inpatient glucose control: a glycemic survey of 126 U.S. hospitals. J Hosp Med 2009;4(9):E7–14.

4. McDermott, K and Roemer, M. Most frequent principal diagnosis for inpatient hospital stays in U.S. hospitals, 2018. Healthcare cost and utilization project. Statistical Brief #227, 2021.

5. Umpierrez GE, Isaacs SD, Bazargan N, et al. Hyperglycemia: an independent marker of in-hospital mortality in patients with undiagnosed diabetes. J Clin Endocrinol Metab 2002;87(3):978–82.

6. American Diabetes Association. Standards of medical care in diabetes: 2024. Diabetes Care 2024;47:S295–306.

7. Korytkowski M, Muniyappa R, Antinori-Lent K, et al. Management of hyperglycemia in hospitalized adult patients in non-critical care settings: an endocrine society clinical practice guideline. J Clin Endocrinol Metab 2022;107(8):2101–28.

8. Finfer S, Chittock DR, Su SY, et al. Intensive versus conventional glucose control in critically ill patients. N Engl J Med 2009;360:1283–97.

9. Fong AC, Cheung NW. The high incidence of steroid-induced hyperglycaemia in hospital. Diabetes Res Clin Pract 2013;99(3):277–80.

Training Hospital Nurses to be Diabetes Champions

Tina Wynn, RD, LD, CDCES

KEYWORDS

- Diabetes • Diabetes champion • Hospital • Diabetes education • Nurse training
- Nursing • Hyperglycemia • Hypoglycemia

KEY POINTS

- Surveys show most hospitals lack enough Diabetes Care and Education Specialists. Programs that have diabetes champions have shown improved glycemic management.
- Diabetes champions can assist with inpatient glycemic management and assistance with patient education including diabetes self-management and survival skills, medication administration, glucose monitoring, and treatment of hypoglycemia.
- Champions can also assist with meeting goals for the American Diabetes Association inpatient diabetes recognition program by performing audits regularly and perform staff education to keep nursing up to date.

INTRODUCTION

Per the Association of Diabetes Care and Education Specialists (ADCES), a Diabetes Care and Education Specialist (DCES) is a health professional who possesses comprehensive knowledge of and experience in diabetes prevention, prediabetes, and diabetes management.[1] In the hospital setting, a health care provider with this specialty can provide in-depth education with patients who have diabetes and help prepare them for how to manage their disease after hospital discharge. Many articles speak to the benefit of hospital outcomes with a DCES including "reduced length of stay, readmission rates, emergency room visits, improved medication adherence, and improved A1c, especially with ranges above 9%, hypoglycemia, and hyperglycemia during and after discharge. In addition, decreased cost of care, fewer after-hour calls, reduced in-hospital medication errors, and increased patient knowledge and satisfaction."[2,3] And though the ADCES reported that the number of DCES who work in the inpatient setting has grown from 21% to 23.8%,[4] there still is a lack of DCES available in most hospital settings to properly serve the critical care and inpatient population.

Endocrine Neoplasia and Hormonal Disorders Department, The University of Texas MD Anderson Cancer Center, 1515 Holcomb Boulevard, Houston, TX 77030, USA
E-mail address: tmwynn@mdanderson.org

Crit Care Nurs Clin N Am 37 (2025) 11–18
https://doi.org/10.1016/j.cnc.2024.08.001
0899-5885/25/© 2024 Elsevier Inc. All rights reserved, including those for text and data mining, AI training, and similar technologies.
ccnursing.theclinics.com

Hospital structures vary on how many DCES are available. In a 2021 survey for ADCES showed 40% of the respondents reported being the only DCES available in the organization, and a quarter of DCESs responded that they work within an interdisciplinary diabetes-focused team.[2]

"There are currently not enough DCESs to meet the needs of the diabetes and pre-diabetes population, and this, coupled with the high demands and lack of adequate staffing …, indicates the need for workforce leveraging to address these gaps. Compounding these challenges, survey respondents indicated that up to one-third of people … at risk of diabetes are challenged with securing affordable medications, accessing healthy food, and finding affordable health care coverage."[3]

For example, our current organization for years had one full-time DCES for the entire hospital, including outpatient and inpatient services. We have now grown to 2 full-time educators dedicated to inpatient alone for a 761 bed hospital, and 2 full-time educators for outpatient services. Though even with this growth, it has been difficult to keep up with the need with our inpatient population.

Due to the challenges of having enough DCES on board to accomplish hospital goals, providing proper education to staff to help support these goals can assist greatly. In the inpatient setting, nurses can play a vital role in helping with education. Though as most nursing staff is overwhelmed with the multitude of so many day-to-day tasks, there may be beneficial outcomes in finding specific nurse volunteers to be a diabetes champion. A champion can serve many purposes to help improve patients with diabetes and their overall outcomes in the hospital setting.

A diabetes champion is a health care professional that can help fill in the gap for diabetes management and diabetes education in the hospital. "Both the American Diabetes Association and the Joint Commission have identified the most successful inpatient diabetes programs as those possessing, specific staff education requirements and identified 'program champions.' Specifically, the Joint Commission diabetes champions can also function as program champions in achieving improved inpatient glycemic management."[5]

DISCUSSION

Due to limited staffing of DCES at our current hospital challenges that have been observed has included held-up discharges and/or patients leaving without proper review of medications and how to use those medications. In addition, with staff turnover and continuous need for reeducation, other challenges have been misunderstandings of proper protocol of insulin timing and hyper/hypoglycemia protocols. An initiative was started this past year to recruit diabetes nurse champions to help assist with these challenges, and gaps seen with limited DCES staff. Our population of patients have continued to grow and therefore has seen continued increase in patients with diabetes. The following are guidelines based on this initiative to recruit diabetes champions and steps taken to achieve these goals.

Getting Started

First step recommended to train nurses to be diabetes champions is to get the support of your hospital, and team. Especially those in leadership roles and/or a physician can help be an advocate for diabetes. Having the support of these individuals can help you get the information needed to reach nursing staff. Some hospitals may require the backing of physician to pursue quality improvement initiatives. Start a committee with these members who can help facilitate this process.

At our organization, we developed a committee consisting of one of the Endocrine physicians who specializes in diabetes, a project manager to help facilitate meetings, inpatient diabetes educators, director of nurse education, and diabetes advance practice providers (APPs), such as nurse practitioners or physician assistants. Try to identify who that could be in the current work setting. It does not have to be these exact roles but think about who can be a representative for nursing, and who can be a representative for the diabetes team.

IIt is important to find a representative from the inpatient nursing staff who is familiar with nursing roles, responsibilities and scope of practice. The nursing representative can also be from the nursing education department or nursing leadership. The nursing leader is familiar with the process for patient care from admission to discharge, operating within hospital policy. Developing strong relationships with nurse managers will aid in identifying nurses interested in becoming diabetes champions. The diabetes nurse champions will need to be able to accomplish their usual day-to-day duties in addition to the duties of being a diabetes nurse champion so realistic expectations of the role should be set prior to training the nurse.

Recruiting from the diabetes management team (physicians, Advanced Practice Registered Nurses, Physicians Assistants and Certified Diabetes Care and Education Specialists) is important because they can identify the education needs of patients with diabetes for after discharge. Identifying the diabetes educational needs of the patient assists the diabetes nurse champion with prioritizing patient education. The diabetes management team also assists with providing education to train the diabetes nurse champion and providing educational resources for the diabetes nurse champion to carry out diabetes education with training materials such as written materials and videos.

If your organization has the resources for a project manager, or an administration staff, it can help stay on track and have the team accomplish goals in timely manner. This person can keep track of action items and deadlines.

In a post COVID, video-conferencing era, it may be easier to make most or all meetings virtual, so most people do not have as many issues attending. Insight is particularly important from all these areas, so attendance is key. Meet monthly until goals/expectations are established and you have identified a diabetes champion from selected units.

How to Identify a Champion

Start with a small area of the hospital or just one area of the intensive care unit (ICU), to test the process. Once you find a system that works and is successful then there can be expansion to other areas of the hospital or ICU. With help of nurse leadership or nursing education, communicate to these units to see who is interested in becoming of diabetes champion.

A champion can be any health care member who preferably belongs to a specific unit in the hospital. Ideally and eventually if able to find at least one champion from every unit or ICU, so they can each focus on their own unit and staff. A champion can be a bedside nurse who has expressed passion for diabetes or education, or even looking for way to grow to a leadership position. Through conversations with staff, you may even find that some of these nurses have interest in becoming a DCES. This is a great way to gain those hours of training to become a certified as a DCES. Though sometimes bedside nursing can be busy with multiple tasks at hand, and therefore, a champion could also be someone who already has a leadership role such as a charge nurse or nurse manager who would be present most days of the week. The key is to find those with a passion that show desire to improve glycemic outcomes for patients.

At our current organization, we have had success with focusing on our nurse managers or nurse leadership of the units to be diabetes champions.

Develop Goals and Expectations

Develop goals for what you want the diabetes nurse champions to accomplish and make expectations clear. What is the time commitment and what exactly is the expectation of what they should accomplish?

What exactly is the goal for a nurse diabetes champion to accomplish? They are going to be an advocate and liaison for diabetes team. Those who represent the diabetes management team should come up with a list of action items needed that has been difficult for the team to accomplish on their own. What actions can help improve outcomes in the hospital setting or help fill the gaps of diabetes education? The following are some examples of specific goals and expectations for the diabetes champions.

One initiative implemented at our current institution is that they assist with quality improvement initiatives for diabetes education. Upon admit every patient with preexisting diabetes, diagnosis is presented with a questionnaire, to identify gaps in diabetes education. After completion of questioner, education is completed by nursing to help clarify these gaps. Diabetes champions assist with education with the patient as well as nurses on the unit to help cover these education gaps. The 2024 ADA Standards of Care for patients in the hospital states that there should be an initial evaluation for the type of diabetes when known, A1c should be measured to be evaluated preadmission glycemia, and diabetes self-management knowledge and behaviors should be assessed on admission and diabetes self-management education provided if available.[6]

Champions can assist with patient education if DCES is unable to see patient or is out (weekends, after hours, or there is limited staffing). Challenges observed especially on weekends and after hours in which discharge is being held due to no DCES available, and patient needs training on glucometer teaching. Instead of holding up, discharge education can be completed by the champion or nursing staff who has been trained.

Trainings provided to the diabetes champions can then also be relayed these trainings to larger group of nursing staff especially to their respective units. Having champions can increase the number of staff to assist for larger wide trainings and keeping the units up to date. The 2024 ADA Standards of Care also states that "institutions are encouraged to perform audits regularly to monitor proper use and in state education/training programs to keep staff up to date."[6]

A challenge within our organization is that education is sometimes requested from a DCES last minute and is needed for patient to discharge. Patient is completed all things and ready for discharge, but due to limited staffing, or if after hours or on the weekend, education cannot be there in a timely manner to get them out when they are ready, or even possibly that day. If a patient is needing something less extensive such as glucometer teaching, providing these resources to the diabetes champions and/or floor nurse can help facilitate these lower need educations as to not hold up discharge for the patient. Ideally, education needs to be implemented in a timely manner to avoid this issue. As mentioned prior, it is recommended by the 2024 ADA Standards of Care to evaluate "diabetes self-management knowledge and behaviors should be assessed on admission, and diabetes management education provided."[6]

What to Train

Provide multiple resources for education and training. Education is continuous for staff to help keep up to date on current information. Possible staff turnover also presents a need for continued retraining of new nurse. Once you have a small group selected, try to set up an initial in-service and training with the diabetes champions and record each session that can be played if retraining is needed. This can be taught and completed by DCES or volunteers from the diabetes management team depending on schedules. Hands-on training can be more beneficial, and when working, a smaller group can be accomplished more quickly. According to the goals and expectations that were made decide what these sessions should cover.

If uncertain what to focus trainings on for your diabetes champions, a resource that is a good place to start is the ADCES 7 Self-care Behaviors for People with Diabetes.[7] These 7 self-care behaviors include healthy coping, healthy eating, being active, taking medication, monitoring, reducing risks, and problem-solving.[8]

In addition, to these 7 self-care behaviors, it would be very important to also provide trainings on what to educate patient to get them out safely and effectively transition to outpatient. Per the 2024 ADA Standards of Care for diabetes care in the hospital, "diabetes self-management education should include knowledge and survival skills needed after discharge, such as medication dosing and administration, glucose monitoring, and recognition and treatment of hypoglycemia."[6]

The inpatient DCES focuses on survival skill for the patient, and assessment of how to get them out safely until they can follow up with a provider. The most common educations that we completed at our organization are insulin teaching and monitoring (with a glucometer or continuous glucose monitor). We have a large population of patients who have steroid-induced hyperglycemia and are brand new to process of checking sugars and taking insulin. Our educators try to focus on the most important things that the patient needs to know to handle his/her medication safely at home until he/she can get additional follow-up.

Diabetes champions should also review hypoglycemia protocols, current organization's inpatient blood glucose goals for inpatient. The 2024 ADA Standards of Care states the following recommendations: "Insulin and/or other therapies should be initiated or intensified for treatment of persistent hyperglycemia starting at a threshold of > or = 180 mg/dL (confirmed on 2 occasions within 24 hours) for non-critically ill (non-ICU) individuals."[6]

For critically ill patients in the ICU, it is recommended that "once therapy is initiated a glycemic goal of 140 to 180 mg/dL for most ICU individuals with hyperglycemia. More stringent glycemic goals, such as 110 to 140 mg/dL, may be appropriate for selected critically ill individuals and are acceptable if they can be achieved without significant hypoglycemia."[6]

Monitor glycemic results monthly to report at these committee meetings to check on progress. In addition, reminding nurses to continue to educate patients on their medication and insulin regimen on a daily basis as they are giving it and explain what they are for continued patient education.

Equipment, Materials, and Resources

After trainings, it would be beneficial to have various written or electronic materials available that champions can refer to for reviewing the information and that can keep them up to date. Written material is something that can be easily left on the units or offices where champions work and should be easily accessible. Electronic versions should be available for each printed written material. Check to see if your facility has a shared folder in the computer system where these can be saved in addition to printed copies.

As mentioned prior if utilizing the AADE 7 care behaviors, there are online and pdf versions. Each self-care behavior has a separate patient education handout that can be used for patients and/or training staff. These can be accessed specifically here https://www.adces.org/diabetes-education-dsmes/adces7-self-care-behaviors.   In addition to the 7 self-care behaviors, there are multiple patient education resources available as well.[8]

Creating custom diabetes educational materials may be beneficial because is would meet the specific needs of the population served by the hospital. Most hospitals have policies that they can only give out information within the organization. Check to see what your facility rules are. At our current organization, there was a diabetes education booklet developed to help cover many diabetes education topics. It is colorful, easy to read, has picture instructions, and has been very easy to use in training patients and staff. This has been approved by our patient education department and updated every 3 years.

This can be a time-consuming project up front but serve to save time later on when complete. This can also be customized to the hospitals primary patient population. As mentioned prior, the education materials should at minimum include survival skills, such as medication dosing, how to administer medication, glucose monitoring, and how to treat hypoglycemia.[6]

Videos

Videos for patient education can be beneficial to have on hand that staff can use to educate patients when time is limited. Or these same videos can be used to educate staff. As mentioned prior, during in services with staff, whether in person or video conference, make sure to have a recording of all trainings in case they are needed again to review by staff.

Within our current organization, there is a patient education department that is very helpful in assisting with creating videos based on our educational handouts. They have assisted us in making several patient education videos covering the topics of insulin administration and glucometer teaching. These videos are given to patients to watch while they are in their hospital room and serve as "pre-education" before discussing in person with them. While the nurse and educator are busy, we can provide these to get the education started. These videos can also be used for patient to watch after education if needing a reminder of the information reviewed. They are available in our hospital room TVs and online through the hospital portal so that they can be accessed after discharge.

These videos are also great resources for the diabetes champions and/or floor nurses to also watch if needing refresher on certain education topics.

There may be rules within the facility that educational videos cannot be taken from outside sources and must be within the organization. Check your policies to see what your options are.

Educational Materials Left on the Unit that Are Approved by Your Facility

In addition to written, online, and video materials, consider physical teaching tools to leave for the champions and nursing staff for teaching if needed. These tools may include demonstration insulin pens, and or vials/syringe, or a demonstration glucometer for glucose checks.

Though most education can be provided at bedside as these things are being performed, but home medications may differ from how it is administered inpatient. For instances, most patients use an insulin pen after discharge, versus in the hospital vials and syringes are used. Also, demonstration items may allow patients to perform return demonstration.

In our current practice, we have provided an insulin-teaching kit that includes all items needed for patient or staff education on how to administer insulin with an insulin pen. Each kit includes 2 demonstration insulin pens, about 30 insulin pen needles, alcohol pads, and instructions on how to use kit and maintain infection control guidelines.

Demonstration insulin pens can be ordered through the insulin pen companies. They do not contain insulin, only normal saline, and are for educational purposes only. Insulin pen needles can also be ordered from the insulin pen needle companies, as long as provided only for educational purposes. Both can be ordered online through insulin company Web site, or through a company sales representative.

Ensure to follow your hospital's infection control guidelines if these are used in patient rooms. Also, double-check hospital policy to make sure they are accepted to be left on the units or in manager's office. Find a safe place to keep them that is agreed upon by the entire staff. These are not for patient use, and only for demonstration. Through discussion at our hospital, it was found to be best to bring a little into the room as possible. Just 1 demonstration pen, and 2 pen needles. The pen needles are discarded in sharps container and left in patient room. The demonstration pen must be sani-wiped before going in and after leaving patient room.

In addition, it would be beneficial to provide a take-home glucometer starter kit that can be used for education, but that patient can ultimately take home. Sample glucometer kits can be ordered from various glucometer company brands, as long as being used for educational purposes. Providing a glucometer kit allows the patient to use and practice with and take home the supply until after discharge when they can pick up more glucometer supplies from the pharmacy.

These kits and glucometers can be used to teach staff, as well as provided to the champions to assist with teachings if needed.

SUMMARY

In summary, most hospitals lack the adequate staffing for DCES, to address diabetes in the ICU and/or the inpatient population. An alternative is having various nurses or nurse leaders that can be diabetes champions for these units to help improve glycemic management and outcomes for patient with diabetes and provide diabetes patient education. These can be nurse leaders, or bedside nurses who have a passion for diabetes and process improvement. It is important to get support from nursing leadership, and leadership from the diabetes management team to ensure training can be implemented. In addition, develop goals and expectations for staff ready to pursue this position. Training should include AADE 7 self-care behaviors, diabetes survival skills, and current hospital policies and protocols for diabetes management in the inpatient or ICU setting. Diabetes champions should receive in-person trainings from DCES of diabetes management team. Other resources should also be provided for training and continued education, such as recording of trainings, videos and modules, and written materials. Tools such as insulin pen teaching kits and glucometer kits should also be provided to these champions for training, and to use for patient education. Champions can assist with training the unit staff in addition to providing gaps in diabetes education due to limited staffing from DCES.

CLINICS CARE POINTS

- Surveys have shown that most hospitals lack enough diabetes care and education specialist and even may just have 1 on staff. Programs that have diabetes champions have shown improved glycemic management.[2]

- Champions can assist with inpatient glycemic management and assistance with patient education. Trainings should include diabetes self-management and survival skills, such as medication dosing and administration, glucose monitoring and treatment of hypoglycemia.[6]
- Champions can also assist with ADA standards of performing audits regularly and perform staff education and training programs to keep nursing up to date.[6]

DISCLOSURE

The author has nothing to disclose.

REFERENCES

1. CBDCE- certification board for diabetes care and education. Healthcare providers. 2024. Available at: https://www.cbdce.org/healthcare-providers. Accessed May 22, 2024.
2. Gwen K, Leigh B, Jennifer NC, et al. Development of quality measures for inpatient diabetes care and education specialist: a call to action. J Healthc Qual 2023;45(5): 297–307.
3. Kavookjian J, Bzowyckyj AS, DiNardo MM, et al. Current and emerging trends in diabetes care and education: 2021 National practice and workforce survey. Sci Diabetes Self Manag Care 2022;48(5):307–23.
4. The Association of Diabetes Care and Education Specialist. The role of the diabetes care and education specialist in the hospital setting. Sci Diabetes Self Manag Care 2022;48(3):184–91.
5. Jornsay DL, Garnett ED. Diabetes champions: culture change through education. Diabetes Spectr 2014 Aug;27(3):188–92.
6. American Diabetes Association Professional Practice Committee. 16. Diabetes care in the hospital: standards of care in diabetes—2024. Diabetes Care 2024; 47(Suppl. 1):S295–306.
7. Judy K. Critical care diabetes education: who, what, when, where and why. Crit Care Nurs Clin 2013;25:123–30.
8. The Association of Diabetes Care and Education Specialist. ADCES7 self-care behaviors. 2023. Available at: https://www.adces.org/diabetes-education-dsmes/adces7-self-care-behaviors. Accessed May 22, 2024.

Noninsulin Diabetes Medications in Hospitalized Children and Adolescents

Mili Vakharia, MSN, APRN, FNP-C[a,b],*

KEYWORDS

- Pediatric diabetes • Inpatient • Hyperglycemia • Metformin • GLP-1 agonists
- SGLT-2 inhibitors

KEY POINTS

- Hospitalized youth with diabetes have specific glycemic targets that must be considered when initiating glucose lowering treatments to avoid iatrogenic hypoglycemia.
- Given lack of sufficient safety data, noninsulin medications including metformin, glucagon-like polypeptide 1 receptor agonists, and sodium glucose transporter protein 2 inhibitors have not been Food and Drug Administration approved for use for pediatric patients in an inpatient setting.
- Pediatric patients should receive an individualized approach to glycemic management using an interdisciplinary team. Factors such as the type of pediatric diabetes, oral intake, prolonged fasting, ketonemia, prior home therapies, and so forth must be considered when formulating diabetes care plan including discharge instructions.

INTRODUCTION

Pediatric diabetes consists of many distinct types with important implications for diagnostic considerations and management. Type 1 diabetes mellitus is an insulin-dependent diabetes that results from autoimmune-mediated destruction of the insulin-producing pancreatic beta cells with progressive insulinopenia and hyperglycemia.[1,2] Insulin remains the mainstay treatment of those with type 1 diabetes.

However, type 2 diabetes mellitus is a metabolic, heterogenous disorder characterized by peripheral, hepatic, and adipose tissue insulin resistance leading to hyperglycemia.[3] Its complex pathogenesis consists of both genetic and environmental factors resulting in insulin secretion defect and subsequent insulinopenia.[3] In pediatrics, the

[a] Division of Pediatric Diabetes and Endocrinology, Department of Pediatrics, Baylor College of Medicine, Houston, TX 77030, USA; [b] Texas Children's Hospital, 1020 MS: BCM320, 6621 Fannin Street, Houston, TX, USA
* Texas Children's Hospital, 1020 MS: BCM320, 6621 Fannin St, Houston, TX.
E-mail address: mili.vakharia@bcm.edu

Crit Care Nurs Clin N Am 37 (2025) 19–33
https://doi.org/10.1016/j.cnc.2024.08.006   ccnursing.theclinics.com
0899-5885/25/© 2024 Elsevier Inc. All rights reserved, including those for text and data mining, AI training, and similar technologies.

medication options for managing type 2 diabetes have evolved over the course of years with oldest known metformin to now newer agents available glucagon-like poly-peptide 1 (GLP-1) receptor agonists and sodium glucose transporter protein 2 (SGLT-2) inhibitors.[3]

Maturity onset diabetes of youth (MODY) is a group of monogenic disorders that causes dysfunction in glucose sensing or insulin production. It is autosomal domi-nantly inherited with 14 genetic mutations identified and makes up about 1% to 5% of pediatric diabetes cases.[4,5] Sulfonylureas are often used for certain MODY types based on genetic mutation. Additionally, less common forms of diabetes in youth include medication-induced diabetes, neonatal diabetes, and mitochondrial diabetes that necessitate specific diagnostic and treatment considerations in the context of their clinical setting.[2]

Use of noninsulin medications in pediatrics is limited to primarily ambulatory care settings. Much of the literature is often extrapolated from adults given limited findings in pediatrics. This article focuses on noninsulin medication management of children and adolescents presenting with hyperglycemia in acute care settings, both critically and noncritically ill.

GLYCEMIC CONSIDERATIONS

In inpatient setting, hyperglycemia is commonly defined as blood glucose level of 140 mg/dL or greater for patients with or without prior diagnosis of diabetes.[6] Histor-ically, stringent glycemic targets of 80 to 110 mg/dL were required to reduce mortality and prevent risks associated with hyperglycemia such as cardiovascular morbidity, poor wound healing, nosocomial infections, delays in surgical procedures, and pro-longed length of hospitalization.[7-9] Hyperglycemia in pediatric populations has been equally associated with increased length of hospital stay and mortality rates reaching as high as 15.2%.[10,11] It is also noted to be an independent risk factor for organ failure and death.[12]

Hypoglycemia remains as rate-limiting step in managing patients with diabetes pre-senting to hospital with hyperglycemia. It is one of the most common iatrogenic compli-cation arising from aggressively lowering glucose levels to maintain normoglycemia.[13] Recent American Diabetes Association (ADA) guidelines recommend a blood glucose target of 140 to 180 mg/dL for patients admitted with hyperglycemia.[14] The more relaxed therapy goals have been derived from the multinational, Normoglycemia in Intensive Care Evaluation-Survival Using Glucose Algorithm Regulation (NICE-SUGAR) trial.[6] The NICE-SUGAR trial demonstrated a significant increased rate in mortality rates by 27.5% versus 25% at 90 days with intensive glucose control ($P = .02$).[15]

Findings from NICE-SUGAR trial showed a 10 to 15 fold greater rates of hypoglycemia in intensively treated patients.[15] Analyses of NICE-SUGAR trial also re-ported that there are wide fluctuations in glucose levels among patients with acute illness and a "fall back" approach must be utilized to avoid prolonged hyperglycemia or hypoglycemia episodes.[15,16] Several other adult-based studies have also shown increased mortality with strict glycemic management (ie, 80–110 mg/dL) in compari-son to less aggressive glucose control (ie, goal of 180 mg/dL).[17-19] It is recommended that for critically ill patients, the target glucose levels of 110 to 140 mg/dL may be applied if there are no concerns for significant hypoglycemia and continuous glucose monitors in an inpatient setting are suggested to avoid hypoglycemia.[8,13]

In pediatrics, several studies have investigated outcomes in critically ill children with intensive glycemic control compared to conventional control and found no advan-tages with tight control.[20-23] The authors in The Control of Hyperglycemia in Pediatric

---

Table 1
American Diabetes Association diagnostic criteria for all types of diabetes in children and adolescents

Diabetes Diagnosis

FPG ≥126 mg/dL (7.0 mmol/L). Fasting is defined as no caloric intake for at least 8 h *or*

2 h PG ≥200 mg/dL (11.1 mmol/L) during OGTT. The test should be performed as described by the World Health Organization, using a glucose load containing the equivalent of 75 g anhydrous glucose dissolved in water * *or*

Hemoglobin A1C (A1C) ≥6.5% (48 mmol/mol). The test should be performed in a laboratory using a method that is NGSP certified and standardized to the DCCT assay * *or*

In a patient with classic symptoms of hyperglycemia or hyperglycemic crisis, a random plasma glucose level of ≥200 mg/dL (11.1 mmol/L)

Diabetes Type Specific, Additional Key Criteria

Type 1	Type 2	MODY
At least 1 positive antibody status: Insulin autoantibody, zinc -transporter 8, glutamic acid decarboxylase, or islet cell antibodies	Negative antibodies Presence of insulin resistance/other risk factors (ie, acanthosis nigricans, hypertension, polycystic ovaries, dyslipidemia, and obesity/overweight)	Hemoglobin a1c <7.5% One parent with diabetes One or more following features specific monogenic cause including renal cysts, partial lipodystrophy, maternally inherited deafness, and severe insulin resistance in the absence of obesity), and monogenic diabetes Prediction model probability >5%

Abbreviations: FPG, fasting plasma glucose; NGSP, National glycohemoglobin standardization program; OGTT, oral glucose tolerance test.
* According to ADA, the diabetes diagnosis requires two abnormal test results from the same sample or in two separate test samples.
Data from Ref.[1,25]

Intensive Care trial evaluated outcomes of 1369 children in 16 intensive care units, who were randomized to target blood glucose range of 72 to 126 mg/dL, or conventional glycemic control, with a target level of less than 216 mg/dL.[20] Their primary outcomes were the number of days alive and free from mechanical ventilation.[20] They found significantly increased episodes of severe hypoglycemia (7.3% vs 1.5%, $P < .001$) in the tight glycemic control group compared to conventional group and found no difference in mortality and ventilator-free days between groups.[20]

In neonates, who have higher propensity for hyperglycemia and hypoglycemia, the latter is far more dangerous contributing to long-term neurologic damage if levels fall below 40 mg/dL.[16] As such, hyperglycemia in this cohort of patients is considered neuroprotective against hypoxia-induced periventricular leukomalacia.[16] Given the physiologic differences in children compared to adults, the adult literature cannot be entirely extrapolated and the differences such as premature physiology must be taken into account.

Therefore, the consensus guidelines derived from several studies and organizations including American Association of Clinical Endocrinology cautions against the use of tight glycemic control in critically ill with or without diabetes and recommended target glucose control in pediatrics as well as adults is 140 to 180 mg/dL.[8,13] For pediatric patients undergoing surgery, International Society for Pediatric Diabetes recommends blood glucose levels of 90 to 200 mg/dL intraoperatively and 140 to 200 mg/dL in the postoperative period.[24]

MEDICAL CONSIDERATIONS IN HOSPITALIZED CHILDREN AND ADOLESCENTS

The ADA has specific management guidelines and diagnostic criteria for all types of diabetes in youth, as described in **Table 1** followed by additional testing that includes autoimmune laboratories to differentiate between type 1 and type 2 diabetes.[3,25] In those with confirmed type 1 diabetes, insulin remains as the only treatment using basal and bolus regimen to mimic pancreatic function.[26]

The findings of the landmark Diabetes Control and Complications Trial (DCCT) study showed significant long-term benefits of multidose insulin regimen compared with traditional once or twice daily insulin therapies.[27] The trial demonstrated the positive correlation between decreased microvascular complications and tight glycemic control. The average starting dose for insulin in child ranges from 0.5 to 1 unit/kg/d with 50% of total daily dose as basal insulin and rest 50% as bolus insulin for meals and hyperglycemia correction.[2]

The ADA position statement on youth presenting with new onset type 2 diabetes recommends initiating metformin along with basal insulin therapy in those with marked hyperglycemia including hemoglobin A1C levels (A1C) greater than 8.5%.[1,3] Metformin is the initial treatment option if hemoglobin A1C levels are less than 8.5% and renal function is normal. In the presence of ketosis or ketoacidosis, insulin must be a pharmacologic option of choice to prevent further metabolic derangement. If hemoglobin A1C goals are not being met, then the use of noninsulin medications must be escalated prior to intensifying insulin regimen.[1]

Table 2 summarizes Food and Drug Administration (FDA)-approved noninsulin medications for pediatrics including GLP-1 agonists and SGLT-2 inhibitors. The findings of Type 2 Diabetes in Youth study showed substantial risk of treatment failure greater than 50% with metformin alone in youth with type 2 diabetes and that aggressive management is required soon after diagnosis.[28]

Current diabetes guidelines recommend initiating basal and correction insulin regimen for patients with type 2 diabetes with poor nutritional intake and in those undergoing surgery.[6] Oral medications such as sulfonylureas should be withheld in patients with poor nutritional intake.[29] Per ADA, continuous intravenous insulin infusion should be utilized for patients in critical care settings to achieve glycemic goals while preventing the risk of hypoglycemia.[14] Those noncritically ill, insulin remains the preferred treatment choice for managing hyperglycemia in the hospital. Oral or other antidiabetic medications can be restarted using hospital discharge protocol that provides guidance on resuming the medication such as 48 to 72 hours after discharge.[14]

Outside of hypoglycemia, other barriers to attaining glycemic control have been identified in hospitalized patients. The hospital course may be complicated by "nothing by mouth" orders for procedures; drug–drug interactions with different medication regimens like glucocorticoids; variability in provider or staff knowledge regarding hyperglycemia and hypoglycemia management; inadequate discharge planning; and stress induced from acute illness worsening hyperglycemia along with renal function.[9] These factors must be considered when initiating pharmacologic treatment of pediatric diabetes.[26]

Hospital discharge planning is also critical to ensuring safety protocols are in place for diabetes management including[9]

- Antihyperglycemic prescription checks prior to discharge
- Coordination of follow-up visits prior to discharge
- Multidisciplinary-led patient education on medical nutrition therapy, self-glucose monitoring, and medication changes such as start of new or resumption of old regimen

Table 2
Noninsulin antihyperglycemic medications for type 2 diabetes in ≥10 y

Medication Name	Class	Mechanism of Action	Dosing	Side Effects, *Contraindications
Metformin hydrochloride (Glucophage, Darmstadt, Germany or Riomet*) *liquid formulation	Biguanide	Reduces hepatic glucose production by decreasing gluconeogenesis and by stimulating peripheral glucose uptake	*Oral Week 1: 500 mg daily Week 2: 1000 mg daily Week 3: 1500 mg daily Week 4: 2000 mg daily	Diarrhea, nausea, vomiting, flatulence, and upset stomach *Warning: lactic acidosis, renal impairment, hypoxic states, excessive alcohol intake hepatic impairment, low vit D, low B12 levels, and hypoglycemia *Severe renal impairment Hypersensitivity Acute or chronic metabolic acidosis, DKA
Liraglutide (Victoza, Plainsboro, NJ) Exenatide (Bydureon) Dulaglutide (Trulicity)	GLP-1 Agonist	Stimulates insulin secretion and inhibits glucagon secretion. Slows down gastric emptying. Reduces appetite and improves satiety	*Injectable week 1: 0.6 mg daily Week 2: 1.2 mg daily Week 3: 1.8 mg daily 2 mg weekly Month 1: 0.75 weekly Month 2: 1.5 mg weekly If ≥18 y, can increase to 3 mg weekly × 1 mo, then 4.5 mg weekly	Nausea, diarrhea, vomiting, constipation, decreased appetite, dyspepsia, constipation, immunogenicity (urticaria), and headache *Warning: Thyroid c-cell tumor, pancreatitis, renal impairment, acute kidney injury, gall bladder disease, hypersensitivity, and hypoglycemia
Empaglifozin (Jardiance, Ridgefield, CT)	SGLT-2 Inhibitors	Targets the SGLT-2 protein expressed in the renal proximal tubule and reduces the reabsorption of sodium and glucose	10 mg daily 25 mg daily	UTI and female genital mycotic infections *Warning: Euglycemic ketoacidosis, volume depletion, urosepsis and pyelonephritis, hypoglycemia, necrotizing fasciitis of perineum

(continued on next page)

Table 2
(continued)

Medication Name	Class	Mechanism of Action	Dosing	Side Effects, *Contraindications
Empaglifozin and metformin hydrochloride (Synjardy)	SGLT-2 inhibitor + metformin	Combination therapy	5 mg empagliflozin/500 mg metformin bid 5 mg empagliflozin/1000 mg metformin bid 12.5 mg empagliflozin/ 500 mg metformin bid 12.5 mg empagliflozin/ 1000 mg metformin bid	UTI and female genital mycotic infections with empagliflozin Diarrhea, nausea, vomiting, flatulence, abdominal discomfort, indigestion, asthenia, and headache with metformin hydrochloride * Renal impairment/failure, dialysis Metabolic acidosis, diabetic ketoacidosis. Hypersensitivity reaction

Data from Ref.[30–33]

NONINSULIN MEDICATIONS
Metformin

For the past several decades, metformin is the most commonly used noninsulin medication and first-line agent for the treatment of type 2 diabetes in pediatrics.[30-32] Metformin has shown improvement in both hemoglobin A1C levels ranging from 1% to 2% and enhanced insulin sensitivity while delaying beta cell decline.[33,34] The dose of metformin is slowly increased and extended-release formulations are used to overcome the gastrointestinal side effects. Baseline renal and liver function must be assessed prior to initiating metformin therapy.[33]

Published clinical consensus guidelines recommend against the use of metformin in hospitalized patients due to potential risk of lactic acidosis, particularly in patients with glomerular filtration rate is 30 to 45 mL/min/1.73 m^2 and other adverse effects.[3,6,14,35,36] In addition, metformin should not be prescribed in patients at risk for cardiac or respiratory insufficiency, dehydration, hepatic impairment including renal failure, renal failure, hypoxia, sepsis, and alcoholism.[3,9,33,35,37]

For patients using radiographic contrast or undergoing surgery, metformin must be discontinued the day prior to procedure and restarted 48 hours after procedure.[9,14] Metformin-associated lactic acidosis (MALA) is a rare complication of metformin use in inpatients and is defined with pH less than 7.35 and lactate greater than 5.0 mmol/L with mortality rate greater than 50%.[38] It is more likely to occur in setting of acute or chronic illness such as renal injury, hepatic/heart failure, shock, or overdose.

Patients with renal impairment from dehydration, surgery, or acute illness have reduced glomerular filtration rates leading to increased plasma metformin levels, especially if metformin intake is continued. As such, the recommendation is to restart only after renal function is stabilized.[38] It would be prudent to consult nephrology specialists if there is persistent renal injury or altered function when attempting to reinstitute metformin. Utility of glucose-lowering agents such as metformin have been trialed in few pediatric and adults studies; however, the general consensus remains against its use given uncertain risks including that of lactic acidosis (**Table 3**).

Glucagon-like Polypeptide 1 Agonists

Glucagon-like polypeptide 1 (GLP-1) receptor agonists have changed the treatment paradigm in pediatric patients with type 2 diabetes given the benefits of weight loss, minimizing hypoglycemia, improving cardiovascular outcomes, and preventing diabetic nephropathy.[6,33] The function of GLP-1 receptor agonist is to mimic the gut-derived incretin hormone GLP-1 and thereby facilitate glucose-stimulated insulin secretion after meals to lower plasma glucose levels.[33] Additional multiple biologic properties of GLP-1 receptor agonists include delayed gastric emptying and central appetite suppression to promote satiety while reducing both food intake as well as food reward signals, contributing to weight loss.[30]

Daily injectable liraglutide, weekly injectables exenatide and dulaglutide were recently approved in pediatric patients with type 2 diabetes. The Evaluation of Liraglutide in Pediatrics With Diabetes (Elipse) trial is a landmark study for GLP-1 receptor agonist, liraglutide in youth onset type 2 diabetes that demonstrated therapeutic benefit of lowering hemoglobin A1C levels of 1% and 1.5% at 26 and 52 weeks, respectively, along with decrease in BMI z-score.[39] However, there are adverse effects such as acute pancreatitis, necrotizing pancreatitis, acute gallbladder disease including cholecystitis have been reported.[32,40] Of note, literature reports that the risk of pancreatitis remains low based on more recent clinical trials.[41-43]

Table 3
Inpatient metformin usage in hospitalized children versus adults

Study	Subjects	Findings
Lacher et al,[56] 2005	15 y old girl	Case report on severe metformin intoxication with lactic acidosis as attempt to commit suicide. Despite hemodialysis, patient continued to have elevated lactate levels with creatinine of 2.4 mg/dL with metformin ingestion
Al-Abdwani,[57] 2020	3 y old girl	Case report of patient with history of complex congenital heart disease and previous cardiac surgery who was admitted to PICU for shock and noted to have MALAs while taking therapeutic dose of metformin. Also, had DVT in right ventricle to pulmonary conduit followed by severe HIE with acute renal injury, which later resolved. As part of neuro rehab, metformin trial of 250 mg twice a day was initiated to recruit existing neural stem cells. Patient was noted to have rise in serum lactate, hyperkalemia 12 h after initiation in the setting of pre-existing acute kidney injury that lead to hyperkalemia and dysrhythmia
Theobald et al,[58] 2020	Mean age of 41 y (ranges 19–79 y), 55% women	40 case reports of patients MALA after acute metformin overdose
Kuno et al,[59] 2023	57 y old woman	Case report in patient with T2D on oral vildagliptin, metformin therapy admitted for severe metabolic acidosis and acute renal injury. Noted to have severe lactic acidosis 5 h after overdosing
Schwetz et al,[60] 2017	78 y old woman, 79 y old woman, and 71 y old man	3 case reports of MALA with concurrent euglycemic ketoacidosis. Older adults presenting with euglycemic ketoacidosis triggered by metformin-mediated inhibition of gluconeogenesis Patient 1: pH = 6.89, lactic acid 22 mmol/L, serum ketoacids 7.4 mmol/L, and blood glucose 63 mg/dL on metformin and insulin treatment Patient 2: pH = 6.80, lactic acid 14.7 mmol/L, serum ketoacids 6.4 mmol/L, and blood glucose 76 mg/dL on metformin Patient 3: pH = 7.21, lactic acid 5.9 mmol/L, and serum ketoacids 16 mmol/L and blood glucose 150 mg/dL on metformin, canagliflozin and liraglutide treatment

Abbreviations: HIE, hypoxic ischemic encephalopathy; DVT, deep vein thrombosis; PICU, pediatric intensive care unit; T2D, type 2 diabetes.

In the Liraglutide safety and efficacy in patients with non-alcoholic steatohepatitis (LEAN) study, a 48 week, double-blinded, randomized, placebo-controlled trial administering liraglutide in adults led to resolution of nonalcoholic steatohepatitis in 9 out of

23 (39%) patients and no increased risk for pancreatitis was reported when compared to placebo group.[44] GLP-1 receptor agonists are contraindicated for use in patients with personal or family history of medullary thyroid cancer as rodent studies have reported GLP-1 receptor agonists can activate c-cell hyperplasia and medullary thyroid cancer.[32,40] As such, patients need counseling on potential risk of medullary thyroid cancer, though rare, and to report symptoms such as neck mass, dysphagia, dyspnea, and persistent hoarseness.[32]

However, the use of GLP-1 receptor agonists in an inpatient setting is limited, especially in pediatrics and remains at research level. Fayfman and group[45] conducted a randomized control trial evaluating the safety and efficacy of exenatide alone or in combination with basal insulin in non–critically ill patients with type 2 diabetes. The authors found that although hyperglycemia treatment with short-acting exenatide twice daily along with basal insulin led to improved glucose values in target range ($P = .023$); however, there was an increased rate of gastrointestinal side effects (10% vs 11% vs 2%). There were no differences both in hypoglycemia episodes and in length of stay ($P = .23$).[45]

Polderman and colleagues[46] also investigated the administration of low-dose liraglutide (0.6 mg) the evening prior to surgery in patients undergoing noncardiac surgery with primary outcome being the difference in median glucose levels 1 hour after surgery. The liraglutide group notably had lower median (interquartile range [IQR]) plasma glucose 1 hour postoperatively compared with the insulin infusion and insulin bolus groups. Though liraglutide stabilized glycemic control postoperatively, patients were noted to have significant episodes of nausea ($P = .007$).[46]

Given their mechanism of action, GLP-1 receptor agonists are associated with adverse effects such as nausea and vomiting with delayed gastric emptying. In general, the published data recommend avoiding the use of GLP-1 receptor agonist in hospitalized children with acute illnesses, including pancreatitis and decreased nutritional intake. The American Society of Anesthesiologists Task Force on Preoperative Fasting recommends withholding daily injectable GLP-1 agonist day prior to surgery and weekly GLP-1 receptor agonist week prior to surgery or procedure to prevent the risk of gastric regurgitation and pulmonary aspiration of gastric contents.[14,47]

Sodium Glucose Transporter Protein 2 Inhibitors

Sodium glucose transporter protein 2 (SGLT-2) inhibitors have been extensively used in adult medicine for managing type 2 diabetes. It maintains glycemic control through promoting urinary glucose excretion while increasing rates of gluconeogenesis and ketosis.[34] In June 2023, empagliflozin became the first SGLT-2 inhibitor to receive FDA approval for use in children and adolescents with type 2 diabetes.[34,48] diabetes study of linagliptin and empagliflozin in children and adolescents (DINAMO) trial, a multicenter study showed reduction in hemoglobin A1C of 0.8% to 1%, similar to their counterpart GLP-1 agonists.[48] In adults, SGLT-2 inhibitors have FDA approval for their use to reduce the risk of major adverse cardiovascular events in those with type 2 diabetes as well as for reducing the risk of glomerular filtration rate decline in those with chronic kidney disease.[32]

According to ADA, SGLT-2 inhibitors can be initiated for hospitalized patients with type 2 diabetes, admitted with heart failure with presumption that there are no contraindications such as presence of severe illness, ketonemia, ketonuria, prolonged fasting or impending surgical procedure.[14] There is scarcity of pediatric data on its effects on cardiovascular function and renal disease that is notably seen with adults.[34] SGLT-2 inhibitors must be discontinued 72 hours before scheduled procedures or surgeries.[14]

There are several adverse effects associated with SGLT-2 inhibitors including genital infections, urinary tract infection, and increased 3 fold risk of diabetic ketoacidosis (DKA), especially in hospital and perioperative settings.[6,32,49] This risk is notably the highest in canagliflozin, followed by empagliflozin and dapagliflozin.[32] On the contrary, there are few pilot randomized controlled studies that have investigated the safety and efficacy of empagliflozin in patients hospitalized with acutely decompensated heart failure in majority of those patients with and without diabetes.[50] In this trial, the authors found that the treatment with empagliflozin was beneficial in increasing urinary output and preventing worsening of heart failure as well as it had no effect on dyspnea scores, length of stay, diuretic response, or N-terminal probrain natriuretic peptide.[50]

Another study compared outcomes of hospitalized patients using SGLT-2 inhibitors and dipeptidyl peptidase 4 inhibitors and found statistically significant similar glycemic effects with no significant increase in hypoglycemia, ketonemia, or lower bicarbonate levels.[51] Given the uncertain and controversial safety concerns with SGLT-2 inhibitors in hospitalized patients, its benefit cannot be assured for use in hospitalized patients, particularly those with multiple comorbidities.[52]

Sulfonylureas

In pediatrics, the class of sulfonylureas has been approved for MODY diabetes types as they facilitate glucose stimulated insulin secretion to improve glycemic control.[5,53] Depending on the MODY subtypes, sulfonylureas such as glyburide are considered first-line agent. However, the use of this class of medications is limited in hospitalized patients due to concerns for hypoglycemia.[9] Deusenberry and colleagues[54] investigated the initiation of sulfonylureas in hospital patients, including those with older age, renal failure, and/or ones using concurrent insulin therapy. Up to 19% of hospitalized patients taking sulfonylureas were noted to have at least one episode of hypoglycemia, with those taking glyburide.[54]

In another retrospective study of 11 acute hospitals in United Kingdom, 30% of patients were found to have hypoglycemia associated with sulfonylureas especially with many experiencing hypoglycemic episodes in overnight and early morning hours.[55] There is paucity of pediatric literature on use of secretagogues like sulfonylureas during hospitalization. Despite the benefits of glucose-lowering effects, the adverse effects of hypoglycemia caused by sulfonylureas are more frequent and severe. The United States scientific societal guidelines recommend against using sulfonylureas for hospitalized patients.[6]

SUMMARY

The safety and efficacy of noninsulin antihyperglycemic agents in the hospital setting remains fully unclear. The data from published trials and consensus guidelines from several scientific societies inform best practices for care of hospitalized children admitted with hyperglycemia. In the vulnerable pediatric population, clinical factors (eg, renal or hepatic insufficiency) must be considered while managing diabetes in critical or noncritical settings and ensure that insulin therapy remains as mainstay of treatment.

Despite the newly available noninsulin medications, such as GLP-1 receptor agonists, SGLT-2 inhibitors, and so forth, it is premature to recommend their usage in an inpatient setting due to significant adverse effects. Larger pediatric prospective studies are needed to determine the utility of noninsulin medications in this cohort of patients in hospital or intraoperative settings. In addition, multidisciplinary diabetes care teams including endocrinologists, intensivists, nurse practitioners, nephrologists, dieticians, physicians' assistants, pharmacists, nurses, and diabetes care and education specialists must be implemented to optimize diabetes care and promote safe discharge.

CLINICS CARE POINTS

- Metformin should be held a day prior to surgical procedure and during acute hospitalization due to risk of lactic acidosis.
- GLP-1 receptor agonist should be discontinued if there are concerns for pancreatitis and 1 to 7 days prior to surgery, depending on weekly versus daily medication, given concerns for delayed gastric emptying as well as potential aspiration in perioperative period.
- In acute illness, SGLT-2 inhibitors are avoided to prevent the risk of DKA and recommended to hold the medication 3 days prior to surgery.

ACKNOWLEDGMENTS

The author would like to acknowledge Celia Levesque (C.V.), NP-C for conceptualizing this topic and providing the opportunity to write this article. Mili Vakharia (M.V.) reviewed the existing literature, drafted the initial article, and revised it. Celia Levesque is the main editor for the article series and has critically reviewed this article as well. M.V. takes accountability for the article being submitted. All authors were actively involved in the discussion for this project and take accountability for the article being submitted.

DISCLOSURE

The author received no funding/financial support for this project and has no conflicts of interest to report. Guarantor statement: M.V. is the guarantor of this study and takes responsibility for the integrity of the data as well as accuracy of the data analysis.

REFERENCES

1. American Diabetes Association Professional Practice Committee; 14. Children and adolescents: *Standards of Care in diabetes—2024*. Diabetes Care 2024; 47(Supplement_1):S258–81.
2. Kharode I, Coppedge E, Antal Z. Care of children and adolescents with diabetes mellitus and hyperglycemia in the inpatient setting. Current Diabetes Report 2019;19:85.
3. Shah AS, Zeitler PS, Wong J, et al. ISPAD clinical practice consensus guidelines 2022: type 2 diabetes in children and adolescents. Pediatr Diabetes 2022;23(7): 872–902.
4. Hoffman LS, Fox TJ, Anastasopoulou C, et al. Maturity onset diabetes in the Young. [Updated 2023 Aug 14]. In: StatPearls [Internet]. Treasure Island (FL): StatPearls Publishing; 2024. Available at: https://www.ncbi.nlm.nih.gov/books/NBK532900/.
5. Greeley SAW, Polak M, Njølstad PR, et al. ISPAD Clinical Practice Consensus Guidelines 2022: the diagnosis and management of monogenic diabetes in children and adolescents. Pediatr Diabetes 2022;23(8):1188–211.

6. Galindo RJ, Dhatariya K, Gomez-Peralta F, et al. Safety and efficacy of inpatient diabetes management with non-insulin agents: an overview of international practices. Curr Diabetes Rep 2022;22(6):237–46.
7. van den Berghe G, Wouters P, Weekers F, et al. Intensive insulin therapy in critically ill patients. N Engl J Med 2001;345(19):1359–67.
8. Blonde L, Umpierrez GE, Reddy SS, et al. American association of clinical Endocrinology clinical practice guideline: developing a diabetes mellitus comprehensive care plan-2022 update. Endocr Pract 2022;28(10):923–1049.
9. Kodner C, Anderson L, Pohlgeers K. Glucose management in hospitalized patients. Am Fam Physician 2017;96(10):648–54.
10. Wintergerst KA, Buckingham B, Gandrud L, et al. Association of hypoglycemia, hyperglycemia, and glucose variability with morbidity and death in the pediatric intensive care unit. Pediatrics 2016;118(1):173–9.
11. Srinivasan V. Stress hyperglycemia in pediatric critical illness: the intensive care unit adds to the stress. J Diabetes Sci Technol 2012;6(1):37–47.
12. Yung M, Wilkins B, Norton L, et al, Paediatric Study Group, & Australian and New Zealand Intensive Care Society. Glucose control, organ failure, and mortality in pediatric intensive care. Pediatr Crit Care Med 2008;9(2):147–52.
13. Apsan J, Sarhis J, Nwosu BU. Inpatient management of children and adolescents with diabetes mellitus. In: Schulman-Rosenbaum RC, editor. Diabetes management in hospitalized patients. *Contemporary Endocrinology.* Cham: Springer; 2023.
14. American Diabetes Association Professional Practice Committee; 16. Diabetes care in the hospital: *Standards of Care in diabetes—2024.* Diabetes Care 2024;47(Supplement_1):S295–306.
15. Finfer S, Chittock DR, Su SY, et al, NICE-SUGAR Study Investigators. Intensive versus conventional glucose control in critically ill patients. N Engl J Med 2009; 360(13):1283–97.
16. Forbes NC, Anders N. Does tight glycemic control improve outcomes in pediatric patients undergoing surgery and/or those with critical illness? Int J Gen Med 2013;7:1–11.
17. Kansagara D, Fu R, Freeman M, et al. Intensive insulin therapy in hospitalized patients: a systematic review. Ann Intern Med 2011;154(4):268–82.
18. Wiener RS, Wiener DC, Larson RJ. Benefits and risks of tight glucose control in critically ill adults: a meta-analysis [published correction appears in JAMA. 2009; 301(9):936]. JAMA 2008;300(8):933–44.
19. Wesorick D, O'Malley C, Rushakoff R, et al. Management of diabetes and hyperglycemia in the hospital: a practical guide to subcutaneous insulin use in the non-critically ill, adult patient. J Hosp Med 2008;3(5 Suppl):17–28.
20. Macrae D, Grieve R, Allen E, et al. A randomized trial of hyperglycemic control in pediatric intensive care. N Engl J Med 2014;370(2):107–18.
21. Agus MS, Wypij D, Hirshberg EL, et al, HALF-PINT Study Investigators and the PALISI Network. Tight glycemic control in critically ill children. N Engl J Med 2017;376(8):729–41.
22. Agus MS, Steil GM, Wypij D, et al. Tight glycemic control versus standard care after pediatric cardiac surgery. N Engl J Med 2012;367(13):1208–19.
23. Vlasselaers D, Milants I, Desmet L, et al. Intensive insulin therapy for patients in paediatric intensive care: a prospective, randomised controlled study. Lancet (London, England) 2009;373(9663):547–56.
24. Jefferies C, Rhodes E, Rachmiel M, et al. ISPAD Clinical Practice Consensus Guidelines 2018: management of children and adolescents with diabetes requiring surgery. Pediatr Diabetes 2018;19(Suppl 27):227–36.

25. American Diabetes Association Professional Practice Committee; 2. Diagnosis and classification of diabetes: *Standards of Care in diabetes—2024*. Diabetes Care 2024;47(Supplement_1):S20–42.

26. Granados A, Iregui AC. Type 1 diabetes management in the hospital setting. Pediatr Rev 2024;45(4):201–9.

27. The Diabetes Control and Complications Trial Research Group. The effect of intensive treatment of diabetes on the development and progression of long-term complications in insulin-dependent diabetes mellitus. N Engl J Med 1993;329:977–86.

28. TODAY Study Group, Bjornstad P, Drews KL, et al. Long-term complications in youth-onset type 2 diabetes. N Engl J Med 2021;385(5):416–26.

29. Sawin G, Shaughnessy A. Glucose control in hospitalized patients. Am Fam Physician 2010;81(9):1121–4.

30. Grøndahl MFG, Johannesen J, Kristensen K, et al. Treatment of type 2 diabetes in children: what are the specific considerations? Expet Opin Pharmacother 2021; 22(16):2127–41.

31. Jensen HK, Rasmussen L, Furu K, et al. Use of non-insulin antidiabetic drugs in children and young adults - a Scandinavian drug utilization study from 2010-2019. Br J Clin Pharmacol 2021;87(11):4470–5.

32. Pinhas-Hamiel O, Zeitler P. Type 2 diabetes in children and adolescents- a focus on diagnosis and treatment. [Updated 2023 Nov 7]. In: Feingold KR, Anawalt B, Blackman MR, et al, editors. Endotext [Internet]. South Dartmouth (MA): MDText.com, Inc.; 2000. Available at: https://www.ncbi.nlm.nih.gov/books/NBK597439/.

33. Van Name MA, Guandalini C, Steffen A, et al. The present and future treatment of pediatric type 2 diabetes. Expet Rev Endocrinol Metabol 2018;13(4):207–12.

34. Krnic N, Sesa V, Mrzljak A, et al. Are treatment options used for adult-onset type 2 diabetes mellitus (equally) available and effective for children and adolescents? World J Diabetes 2024;15(4):623–8.

35. Umpierrez GE, Hellman R, Korytkowski MT, et al. Endocrine Society. Management of hyperglycemia in hospitalized patients in non-critical care setting: an endocrine society clinical practice guideline. J Clin Endocrinol Metab 2012; 97(1):16–38.

36. Moghissi ES, Korytkowski MT, DiNardo M, et al, American Association of Clinical Endocrinologists, & American Diabetes Association. American Association of Clinical Endocrinologists and American Diabetes Association consensus statement on inpatient glycemic control. Diabetes Care 2009;32(6):1119–31.

37. DeFronzo R, Fleming GA, Chen K, et al. Metformin-associated lactic acidosis: current perspectives on causes and risk. Metabolism 2016;65(2):20–9. PMID: 26773926.

38. Dyatlova N, Tobarran NV, Kannan L, et al. Metformin-associated lactic acidosis (MALA) [Updated 2023 Apr 17]. In: StatPearls [Internet]. Treasure Island (FL): StatPearls Publishing; 2024. Available at: https://www.ncbi.nlm.nih.gov/books/NBK580485/.

39. Tamborlane WV, Barrientos-Pérez M, Fainberg U, et al, Ellipse Trial Investigators. Liraglutide in children and adolescents with type 2 diabetes. N Engl J Med 2019; 381(7):637–46.

40. Filippatos TD, Panagiotopoulou TV, Elisaf MS. Adverse effects of GLP-1 receptor agonists. Rev Diabet Stud: Reg Dev Stud 2014;11:202–30.

41. Drucker DJ, Sherman SI, Bergenstal RM, et al. The safety of incretin-based therapies–review of the scientific evidence. J Clin Endocrinol Metab 2011;96(7): 2027–31.

42. Egan AG, Blind E, Dunder K, et al. Pancreatic safety of incretin-based drugs–FDA and EMA assessment. N Engl J Med 2014;370(9):794–7.
43. Nreu B, Dicembrini I, Tinti F, et al. Pancreatitis and pancreatic cancer in patients with type 2 diabetes treated with glucagon-like peptide-1 receptor agonists: an updated meta-analysis of randomized controlled trials. Minerva Endocrinology 2023;48(2):206–13.
44. Armstrong MJ, Barton D, Gaunt P, et al, LEAN trial team. Liraglutide efficacy and action in non-alcoholic steatohepatitis (LEAN): study protocol for a phase II multi-center, double-blinded, randomized, controlled trial. BMJ Open 2013;3(11): e003995.
45. Fayfman M, Galindo RJ, Rubin DJ, et al. A randomized controlled trial on the safety and efficacy of exenatide therapy for the inpatient management of general medicine and surgery patients with type 2 diabetes. Diabetes Care 2019;42(3): 450–6.
46. Polderman JAW, van Steen SCJ, Thiel B, et al. Peri-operative management of patients with type-2 diabetes mellitus undergoing non-cardiac surgery using liraglutide, glucose-insulin-potassium infusion or intravenous insulin bolus regimens: a randomized controlled trial. Anesthesia 2018;73(3):332–9.
47. American Society of Anesthesiologists Committee. Practice guidelines for preoperative fasting and the use of pharmacologic agents to reduce the risk of pulmonary aspiration: application to healthy patients undergoing elective procedures. An updated report by the American Society of Anesthesiologists task force on preoperative fasting and the use of pharmacologic agents to reduce the risk of pulmonary aspiration. Anesthesiology 2017;126:376–93.
48. Laffel LM, Danne T, Klingensmith GJ, et al, DINAMO Study Group. Efficacy and safety of the SGLT2 inhibitor empagliflozin versus placebo and the DPP-4 inhibitor linagliptin versus placebo in young people with type 2 diabetes (DINAMO): a multicenter, randomized, double-blind, parallel group, phase 3 trial. Lancet Diabetes Endocrinol 2023;11(3):169–81.
49. Thiruvenkatarajan V, Meyer EJ, Nanjappa N, et al. Perioperative diabetic ketoacidosis associated with sodium-glucose co- transporter-2 inhibitors: a systematic review. British Journal of Anesthesia 2019;123(1):27–36.
50. Damman K, Beusekamp JC, Boorsma EM, et al. Randomized, double- blind, placebo-controlled, multicenter pilot study on the effects of empagliflozin on clinical outcomes in patients with acute decompensated heart failure (EMPA-RESPONSE-AHF). Eur J Heart Fail 2020;22(4):713–22.
51. Huang W, Whitelaw J, Kishore K, et al. The comparative epidemiology and outcomes of hospitalized patients treated with SGLT2 or DPP4 inhibitors. J Diabetes Complicat 2021;35(12):108052.
52. Koufakis T, Mustafa OG, Ajjan RA, et al. The use of sodium-glucose co-transporter 2 inhibitors in the inpatient setting: is the risk worth taking? J Clin Pharm Therapeut 2020;45(5):883–91.
53. Delvecchio M, Pastore C, Giordano P. Treatment options for MODY patients: a systematic review of literature. Diabetes Therapy 2020;11(8):1667–85.
54. Deusenberry CM, Coley KC, Korytkowski MT, et al. Hypoglycemia in hospitalized patients treated with sulfonylureas. Pharmacotherapy 2012;32(7):613–7.
55. Swanson CM, Potter DJ, Kongable GL, et al. Update on inpatient glycemic control in hospitals in the United States. Endocr Pract 2011;17(6):853–61.
56. Lacher M, Hermanns-Clausen M, Haeffner K, et al. Severe metformin intoxication with lactic acidosis in an adolescent. Eur J Pediatr 2005;164(6):362–5.

57. Al-Abdwani R. Metformin-induced lactic acidosis reported in the youngest pedi-
    atric patient with impaired renal function. Oman Med J 2020;35(4):e162.
58. Theobald J, Schneider J, Cheema N, et al. Time to development of metformin-
    associated lactic acidosis. Clin Toxicol 2020;58(7):758–62.
59. Kuno H, Fujimaru T, Kadota N, et al. Severe lactic acidosis with euglycemic diabetic
    ketoacidosis due to metformin overdose. CEN Case Reports 2023;12(4):408–12.
60. Schwetz V, Eisner F, Schilcher G, et al. Combined metformin-associated lactic
    acidosis and euglycemic ketoacidosis. Wien Klin Wochenschr 2017;129(17–18):
    646–9.

Using Diabetes Technology in Hospitalized Patients

Deborah L. McCrea, EdD, MSN, RN, FNP-BC, CNS, CNE, CEN, CFRN, EMT-P

KEYWORDS

- Insulin pump • Continuous glucose sensor • Analog insulins • Open looping device
- Sensor augmented device • Benefits of intensive insulin management insulin pump/CGM inpatient consensus guidelines
- Establishing an insulin pump/CGM system

KEY POINTS

- There are an estimated 350,000 persons wearing insulin pumps and 2.4 million wearing continuous glucose sensors.
- Technological advantages allow these systems to work together with algorithms to offer more precise delivery of insulin.
- Open loop, sensor augmented, hybrid automatic, fully automated, and do-it-yourself automated delivery merge pump/sensors/algorithms to fine tune delivery/dosage of insulin.
- A multitude of studies and national organizations including The Joint Commission support the use of these devices while in the hospital.

INTRODUCTION

Currently, 700 million people will have been diagnosed with diabetes by 2040.[1] An estimated 38.4 million persons in the United States have diabetes. Over 8 million have not been diagnosed and 97 million have prediabetes. Between 1.2 million and 2 million people have been diagnosed with Type 1 diabetes (T1D) including between 187,000 and 304,000 children and adolescents. Approximately, 12.3% of all people with diabetes (PWD) are using insulin.[2–6]

The landmark 1983 to 1989 Diabetes Control and Complications Trial (DCCT) found persons with T1D who practiced intensive insulin management utilizing either multiple daily injections (MDI) or insulin pump achieved lower hemoglobin A1C levels and had less than 76% retinopathy, 56% nephropathy, and 60% neuropathy. A follow-up study, the Epidemiology of Diabetes Interventions and Complications trial, found 96% of the DCCT participants who practiced intensive insulin therapy over a long period of time did reduce cardiovascular, advanced retinopathy, and neuropathy complications.[7,8]

Department of Graduate Studies, UTHealth Houston, Cizik School of Nursing, 6901 Bertner, Suite 695, Houston, TX 77030, USA
E-mail address: Deborah.L.McCrea@uth.tmc.edu

Crit Care Nurs Clin N Am 37 (2025) 35–52
https://doi.org/10.1016/j.cnc.2024.07.001
0899-5885/25/© 2024 Elsevier Inc. All rights are reserved, including those for text and data mining, AI training, and similar technologies.
ccnursing.theclinics.com

HISTORY OF DIABETES TREATMENT TECHNOLOGY
Insulin Pumps

Prior to 1990, there were less than 7000 pump wearers in the United States. Currently, there are estimates of 350,000 and 400,000 people regardless of the type of diabetes. The first insulin pump was developed in 1963 and was the size of a backpack that injected intravenous (IV) insulin. The 1970s advances in technology allowed development of smaller devices that were used in the research arena. The first subcutaneously "auto-syringe pump was developed and weighed approximately 1 lb. In 1983, Mini-Med developed the first "programmable" pump and newer generation pumps came on the market in the 1990s. As technology improved, Medtronic Diabetes developed the first "intelligent pump" to link glucose meters wirelessly to send glucose reading to the pump so a "bolus wizard" would determine a more precise dose of insulin. It allowed more accurate meal or correction bolusing by using the current glucose and carbohydrate intake, including allowing prolonged bolus patterns based on the type of carbohydrate consumed. It also had the capability of variable basal rates which included altering patterns for a variety of metabolic needs such as dawn phenomena, menstruation, etc.[5,9–17] **Box 1** discusses the clinical indications for insulin pump use.

Analog Insulins

The advancement in insulins analogs allows insulin pumps to better mimic the human pancreas. The first insulins, extracted from canine and bovine pancreases, saved countless lives but caused allergic reactions. In 1978, the first genetically engineered synthetic "human" insulin was made available in 1982. Currently, PWD have more

---

Box 1
Clinical indication for insulin pump use[10,18]

- Frequent multiple daily injections (MDI)
- Inadequate glycemic management despite optimized MDI
- Recurrent unpredictable hypoglycemia or hypoglycemia unawareness
- Nocturnal hypoglycemia
- Dawn phenomenon.
- Preconception planning/pregnancy
- Extreme insulin sensitivity
- Gastroparesis
- Early neuropathy/nephropathy
- Renal transplantation
- Needle phobia
- Erratic schedules
- Frequent travel
- Desire for flexibility
- Inconvenience of MDI
- Adolescents with eating disorders

insulin choices. Better blood glucose management has improved over the decades since analog insulins which have a more predictable insulin action curse came on the market. In addition, advances in insulin pump programming including the use of additional basal and bolus patterns have also help persons with diabetes obtain better diabetes management.[16,19–22] **Table 1** discusses the various analog insulins.

Continuous Glucose Monitor Sensors

Approximately 2.4 million Americans use continuous glucose monitor (CGM) sensors [9] The forerunners to glucose monitoring began during medieval times when glucose testing started with urine examination to help identify various diseases. During the nineteenth century, sugar was discovered in urine and in 1838, sugar was isolated in blood serum. In 1945, self-testing of urine, allowing a chemical reaction using a color chart assess levels. In the late 1950s, reagent strips were developed to test capillary glucose, but was mainly available in hospitals. The first meters with digital display were developed in the 1980s for home use. Over the next 3 decades, meters became more accurate, smaller, required less blood samples, and had memory storage.[6,10,24–26]

Continuous glucose monitor (CGM) sensor prototypes were being developed in the 1970s. The first CGM device for home use was the "GlucoWatch." In 1999, MiniMed developed the first CGM sensor and was used by physicians. A subcutaneous catheter inserted in the physician's office measured interstitial fluid (ISF) glucose levels and was gathered over 3 days. The data are blinded to the patient, and they log events such as food intake, exercise, and insulin dosing. The physician downloaded the data, adjusted doses, and offered teaching to improved glycemic control. In 2004, Medtronic Diabetes, introduced the first patient-use CGM called the Guardian. In 2006, the first integrated diabetes system, linking the insulin pump and CGM was developed and considered an "open loop" system. This was the first development toward the future "closed-looped" insulin delivery system.[13,24–31] **Table 2** lists the current CGM Systems.

INSULIN PUMP AND CONTINUOUS GLUCOSE MONITOR SYSTEM FUNCTION

Over the last 10 years, with the advances in insulin pumps and CGMs, clinicians can now guide a more accurate delivery of insulin with resultant improved glycemic control. Some opt for simplicity of older systems. However, the community of persons living with T1D has embraced multifaceted systems that integrate data involvement from CGM systems and complex algorithms with the development of their own do-it-yourself systems.

Table 1
Analog insulin chart[16,19,23]

Ultra Acting		Rapid Acting		Short Acting	
Generic	Trade name	Generic	Trade Name	Generic	Trade Name
Insulin aspart	Fiasp ®	Insulin lispro	Humalog®	Regular	None
		Insulin lispro	Admelog®		
Insulin lispro aabc	Lyumjev®	Insulin aspart	Novolog ®		
		Insulin glulisine	Apidra®		

Table 2
Manufactures of continuous glucose monitor system and automated insulin delivery system[21,32,33]

Manufacturers	Continuous Glucose Monitor System Model	Automated Insulin Delivery System Integration
Abbot	• Freestyle Libre	• None
	• FreeStyle Libre 2	• None
	• FreeStyle Libre 3	• Coming soon
	• FreeStyle Libre 14-d	• None
	• FreeStyle Libre 2 Plus	• Tandem t:slim × 2
		• Insulet Omnipod 5
	• FreeStyle Libre PRO-HCP tool	• None
Dexcom	• Dexcom G6	• Tandem t:slim x2
		• Insulet Omnimod 5
	• Dexcom G6 PRO- HCP tool	• None
	• Dexcom G7	• Tandem t:slim × 2
		• Beta Bionics iLet
Medtronic Diabetes	• Medtronic Guardian Connect System	• Minimed 670G
		• Minimed 770G
	• Guardian Sensor 3 with Guardian Link 3 transmitter	• Minimed 630G
		• Minimed 770G
	• Guardian 4	• Minimed 780G
Senseonics	• Eversence E3 CGM System	• None

Conventional Insulin Pump Therapy

Current insulin pumps deliver continuous insulin infusion through a subcutaneous small catheter or tubeless patch pump system, most often with ultra rapid or rapid-acting insulins. SEE **Table 3** for list of current insulin pumps in the United States.

There are 2 modes of operation. The basal rate delivers continuous insulin over 24 hours and is programmed to meet basic metabolic needs. Basal dosing is what

Table 3
Manufactures of insulin pumps in the United States, 2024[21,34]

Manufacturers	Pump Model	Web Site, Telephone
CeQur	• CeQur Simplicity Pump Patch	https://myceqursimplicity.com/ 888-552-3787
Beta Bionics	• iLet Bionic Pancreas System	https://www.betabionics.com/ 855-745-3800
Medtronic Diabetes	• MiniMed™ 630G	https://www.medtronicdiabetes.com/ 800-646-4633
	• MiniMed™ 770G	
	• MiniMed™ 780G hybrid closed loop	
Insulet Corp.	• Omnipod 5	https://www.omnipod.com/ 800-591-3455
	• Omnipod Dash	
Tandem Diabetes Care	• t:slim × 2 insulin pump with control-IQ	https://www.tandemdiabetes.com/ 877-801-6901
	• Mobi Insulin patch pump	
Mannkind Corp.	• V-Go patch pump	https://www.go-vgo.com/ 866-881-1209

is required to keep glucose in therapeutic ranges while not eating. The bolus rates are extra insulin needed for carbohydrate intake and hyperglycemia to keep glycemic within targets. Other features can be programmed into the pump based on the person's desire for individual features. This can include setting up special basal rate patterns for travel, menstruation, erratic work schedules, etc. Additional bolus features can be programmed to include extended insulin delivery for certain foods that cause an erratic rise in glucose levels such as foods that have more fat and complex carbohydrates. This feature can also help people who may have gastroparesis, so insulin is delivered slowed down to match their slower digestion rates. As technology evolves, insulin pumps continue to have more "bells and whistles." Currently, pumps are categorized as (1) Conventional insulin pumps, (2) Sensor-Augmented Insulin Pumps (SAP), and (3) Automated Insulin Dosing Systems (AID).[5]

Continuous Glucose Meter Systems

CGM systems utilize a catheter inserted in various subcutaneous areas that measures ISF glucose values. The catheter uses a glucose-oxidase platinum electrode to send glucose levels to a receiver device. Glucose travels between blood vessels to ISF. Fingerstick glucose meters measure capillary blood. CGM measures ISF blood glucose and these are never identical. When glucose is rising in the capillaries, sensor readings will lag. When capillary glucose is dropping, the sensor will be reading higher.[35]

The "real time" CGM collects data every 5-minutes and can show trend arrows to alert rise and fall rates and can allow family to "follow" sensor readings in real time so interventions can be made if incapacitated. Cloud-based programs allow data to be downloaded to view a comprehensive picture of glycemic control.[35] Users are taught if they feel symptoms that do not match the sensor, to always follow up with a fingerstick reading.[5,35–37] **Table 4** shows substances/medications that can alter CGM.

Open Loop Insulin Delivery

The first "open loop system" was developed in 2005 when Medtronic Diabetes developed the Guardian CGM. The user enters their CGM reading and carbohydrates to

Table 4
Continuous glucose monitoring devices interfering substances[35]

Medication	Systems Affected	Effect
Acetaminophen >4 g/day Any dose	Dexcom G6, Dexcom G7 Medtronic Guardian	Higher sensor readings than actual glucose Higher sensor readings than actual glucose
Ascorbic acid (vitamin C), >500 mg/day	FreeStyle Libre 14-d FreeStyle Libre 2 FreeStyle Libre 3	Higher sensor readings than actual glucose
Hydroxyurea	Dexcom G6, Dexcom G7, Medtronic Guardian	Higher sensor readings than actual glucose
Mannitol (IV or as peritoneal dialysis solution)	Senseonics Eversense	Higher sensor readings than actual glucose
Sorbitol (IV or as peritoneal dialysis solution)	Senseonics Eversense	Higher sensor readings than actual glucose

allow the bolus calculator to determine a dose. The person makes a final decision to allow the pump to deliver the insulin.

Sensor-Augmented Insulin Pump

SAPs also known as partial closed-loop systems utilize an insulin pump, CGM, and an algorithm that automates insulin suspension when glucose is low or predicted to go low within the next 30 minutes and automatically shuts off. In 2006, the Medtronic Paradigm REAL-Time was developed as the first SAP. The pump adjusts basal rates when outside the targeted ranges. However, this "non-feedback" system still requires manual adjustments by the pump wearer such as entering carbohydrate amounts. The Tandem X2 Basal IQ and Control IQ, the Medtronic 670G, 770G with Guardian sensor, and non-FDA-approved open-source systems are current options. However, technology is rapidly changing and vendors enter and leave the market quickly.[5,14,35]

Hybrid Automated Insulin Dosing (Also Known as Hybrid Closed Loop)

Hybrid insulin pump system automatically alters basal insulin delivery in response to sensor glucose values. The person still needs to enter mealtime doses manually. Advanced hybrid AID systems are also available now and not only adjust basal insulin delivery but also deliver automatic correction bolus but still require mealtime dosing.[14]

Fully Automated Insulin Dosing vs Delivery Systems

The AID systems, known as closed-loop systems, incorporate an insulin pump, a CGM system, and an algorithm to simulate physiologic insulin delivery and are accomplished by adjusting basal delivery in real time. AID systems require manual entry of carbohydrates consumed to calculate prandial doses.[14,28,35,38–41]

Do-It-Yourself (Also Known as Loop, Looping, OPEN Artificial Pancreas System, Android Artificial Pancreas System)

"Do-it-yourself" AID systems are now available. This system utilizes only certain insulin pumps, CGM systems, plus an open-source algorithm bridging device to communicate through a self-built phone application to allow changing of basal rates automatically, which overrides the normal programming of the pump settings. There are an estimated 2200 PWD worldwide who utilize "Looping Technology" which was started in 2014 from a #WeAreNotWaiting social media group of parents of children with T1DM. The open-source artificial pancreas system (OpenAPS) movement assembled various components such as a mini-computer, radio stick, battery, existing insulin pump, and CGM initially and has evolved from there to more advanced features. Potential benefits include improved time in range, decreased hemoglobin A1C, less lows and high BGs, improved quality of life, and improved sleep. A recent study found persons with T1D using an OpenAPS had significantly higher percentage of time in range glucose targets than those on SAP therapy.[42] Some disadvantages include limited availability of insulin pumps that have remote control abilities, additional hardware needed, ability to "build" the system, resistance of some health care providers (HCP) to support patients with the treatment choice, and liability concerns. The 2024 American Diabetes Association (ADA) standards stated HCP cannot prescribe these devices but can assist in their management.[35,40,42–44]

Artificial Pancreas

Many people call the Full AID system an artificial pancreas (AP); however, the AP does not consider exocrine functions of the pancreas.[26]

Bihormonal (Bionic Pancreas)

AID systems that incorporate 2 hormones such as insulin and glucagon are available. Other combinations are being studied such as insulin and pramlintide.[10,26,45]

BENEFITS OF INTENSIVE INSULIN MANAGEMENT

Advances utilizing device-driven care, advanced pumps, more predictable faster insulins, and CGM systems have demonstrated benefit to both glycemic control, reduction of long-term complications, hypoglycemia, hyperglycemia, and diabetic ketoacidosis compared to the use of MDI. SAPs result in significant improvement in hemoglobin A1C levels, as compared with injection therapy.[35,46]

Recent studies found SAPs and CGMs had improved hemoglobin A1C without an increased rate of hypoglycemia. The SAP therapy for hemoglobin A1C Reduction study looked at SAP and injections in persons with inadequately controlled T1D and found significant improvements in levels.[5,46,47]

Technology then advanced to also add a low-glucose sensor "threshold suspend" delivery system to suspend insulin delivery. "Predictive-threshold suspend" was the next technology shortly afterward that found a 50% to 80% reduction in nighttime hypoglycemia and a 31% to 50% reduction in hypoglycemia when compared to SAP alone.[48–51]

Insulin Pump/Continuous Glucose Monitor Inpatient Consensus Guidelines

Several professional organizations including the Joint Commission Accreditation of Hospital Organizations, Endocrine Society, the American Association of Clinical Endocrinology, the ADA, the Association of Diabetes Care and Education Specialists, and the American College of Endocrinology all support PWD to continue use of insulin pumps/CGM systems while hospitalized if deemed clinically appropriate and under care of diabetes specialist service. They must have cognitive and physical ability, the desire for self-care, and able to follow hospital policies while an inpatient. Policies need to include documentation of pump settings, recommendations of glucose measurements, and signed patient agreements.[5,35,52]

In 2020, The Diabetes Technology Society (DTS) acknowledged the rapid use of diabetes technologies especially while hospitalized. The pandemic increased the realization that diabetes technology can assist health care providers (HCP) to be alerted quickly to hypoglycemia and other events. The FDA provided a policy to allow monitoring of patients more effectively and reduce exposures to certain communicable diseases by allowing the use of personal insulin pumps/CGM systems while hospitalized. CGMs allow less frequent point of care (POC) capillary glucose testing, decreased hyperglycemic episodes, and decreased hypoglycemic episodes.[18,35,37,53,54]

The DTS organized the Continuous Glucose Monitor and Automated Insulin Dosing System in the Hospital Consensus Guideline Panel and developed 77 recommendations to support hospitalized patients with diabetes and met again in 2023 to review progress. See **Box 2**. More expert recommendations for CGM implementation were formulated and can be viewed in their meeting report.[39,55,56]

Topics such as interaction of data with the user, the nursing, pharmacy, electronic health record (EHR), hybrid protocols, combining POC, blood glucose monitoring, and CGM were included.[39] The consensus statement also included the use of AID systems.[5,28,54,55]

In 2021, the Joint Commission published a "Quick Safety" document to guide strategies for HCP to support PWD to continue to use their personal insulin pumps and CGM systems while hospitalized. See **Box 3**. They developed 7 areas based on these requirements. Recommendations included utilizing a multidisciplinary team who

> **Box 2**
> **Diabetes technology society continuous glucose monitor use in hospital panel recommendations topics**
>
> - Nursing issues, protocols, order sets, and education for using continuous glucose monitor (CGM)
> - Implementing CGM programs for use
> - Quality metrics and financial implications
> - CGM in the critical care setting, labor/delivery, and hemodialysis
> - Research session on CGM in the hospital
> - Starting a CGM on hospitalized patients
> - Insulin delivery systems in the hospital
> - CGM in children
> - Data integration for inpatient use and telemetry
> - Accuracy of CGM/comparison with point of care (POC) blood glucose testing
> - Discharge planning with CGM

would consider continency planning with a policy and procedures with following points in mind: (1) patient condition changes and when no longer safe to manage their systems, (2) the availability of batteries if the patient does not have them, (3) availability of replacement medication for the pump, and (4) infusion device fails/damage, rendering it unusable.[55]

The Continuous Glucose Monitor and Automated Insulin Dosing System in the Hospital Consensus Guideline Panel recommended the following potential opportunities for initiation of CGM in the hospital.[56] See **Box 4**.

Box 5 discusses Consensus Panel recommendations for overall practice in the Clinical Practice.

Box 6 discusses Consensus Panel recommendations for special situations of the perioperative period.

Box 7 discusses Consensus Panel recommendations for special situations of pregnancy/delivery.

Box 8 discusses Consensus Panel recommendations for special situations of Emergency Center/ICU.

Box 9 discusses Consensus Panel recommendations for Devices in the Ward.

Box 10 discusses who should keep their pump while in the hospital.

> **Box 3**
> **The Joint Commission recommendations[41,57]**
>
> - Policy and Procedure
> - Home medication use
> - Medication self-administration
> - Orders: Insulin dosages and glucose monitoring frequency
> - Medical record documentation
> - Education of staff, patient, and family
> - Conducting risk assessment

Box 4

Opportunities to for initiation of Insulin pump/continuous glucose monitor in the hospital[5,39,53,56]

- Coronavirus disease-2019 or other isolation situations especially in critical care
- Noncritical illnesses
- No medication interference
- No change in cognitive status
- Not being treated for diabetic ketoacidosis (DKA) or hyperglycemic hyperosmolar syndrome (HHS)
- No concern for pump malfunction
- Surgery less than 2 hours
- No ionizing/magnetic radiation
- Continuation of AID Systems in the hospital
- Improved glycemic outcomes
- Patient satisfaction

The panel recommended the following as contraindications to hospital use of insulin pump/CGM systems. See **Box 11**.

Box 12 discusses the Consensus Panel recommendations as patient responsibilities.

Box 13 discusses the Consensus Panel recommendations for HCP responsibilities.

Box 5

Clinical practice[28,52,53,56]

- Consult with inpatient diabetes team
- Avoid relying on CGM data for glycemic exertions of less than 40 mg/dL or greater than 500 mg/dL
- Avoid use for treatment of DKA or rapidly changing glucose/electrolytes
- Use trend arrows to prevent extreme excursions
- Set alarm thresholds for targets
- Basal insulin or basal plus bolus correction insulin plan is preferred for the noncritical patient with poor oral intake or nothing by mouth.
- Basal, prandial, and correct components is preferred treatment for most noncritically ill with adequate nutritional intake
- Sole use of correction or supplemental insulin without basal insulin (formally called sliding scale) is discouraged
- Daily data review and documentation
- Changing pump supplies and refilling the reservoir
- Capillary glucose measurement and insulin dose adjustments
- Cybersecurity and hospital policies
- Reasons to discontinue the devise(s) including, patient related, hospital related, device related, medication related, nutrition related, surgical related

Box 6
Special situations: perioperative period[28,37,52,53,56–59]

- Ambulatory/short-term surgical procedures for up to 2 to 3 h
- Policy reviewed/signed
- Preop checklist completed
- Review pump settings and adjust as needed
- Bring all pump supplies
- Insert new sites away from surgical area
- Document equipment and inspected for proper function
- Document skin issues or leakage of insulin
- Access to devices to suspend or disconnect
- If insulin pump is discontinued, IV or subcutaneous insulin must be started
- Not recommended if insulin requirements fluctuate significantly intraoperatively '
- AID systems can be continued during operation if no concerns regarding malfunction.
- Some studies on accuracy of CGM with electrocautery

Box 7
Special situations: pregnancy/delivery[28,35,52,60,61]

- CGMs in pregnant persons with T1D can improve maternal and fetal outcomes including (1) time in glycemic range without increase in hypoglycemia, (2) lower large-for-gestational-age babies, (3) fewer neonatal intensive care unit (ICU) admissions, (4) reduced neonatal hypoglycemia, and (5) decreased length of stay (LOS).
- Increase insulin requirement during pregnancy and falls sharply after delivery and breast feeding
- Advise to continue insulin pump/CGM during a hospitalization to identify glucose trends

Box 8
Special situations: devices in the emergency center/intensive care unit[28,37,52,56,58,62]

- Optimal glucose management results in improved outcomes and decreased LOS.
- Continuous IV insulin is most effective in ICU using validated written or computerized protocols
- Optimal for isolated patients who require HCP to frequently don/doff equipment to POC test
- Recommendations for venous/arterial blood to ensure CGM is functioning properly
- Drawbacks is POC is more labor intensive
- CGM data helpful for IV insulin infusion, steroid hyperglycemia, nutrition therapy
- HCP can miss the full 24-h glycemic profile and excursions with only POC testing
- Will not have target alarms available if only POC testing
- Recommendations for hybrid approach with both POC and CGM testing

Box 9
Special situations: devices in the ward[28,37,39,52,54,56,58,62,63]

- High risk of hypoglycemia, then CGM rather than POC alone
- Insulin pump use should continue rather than changing to basal bolus insulin
- CGM detected higher number of hypoglycemic events
- Capillary/serum blood glucose (BG) after procedures recommended for noncritically ill patients
- Better detection of nocturnal event, hypoglycemia unawareness, corticosteroids, various nutrition modalities, and reduced awareness by staff

Box 10
Who should keep their pump?[56,64]

- Surgical procedure less than less than 2 hours
- Admitted to ward in a non-critically ill condition
- Able to operate insulin pump with mentally, physically, and cognitively intact
- Agreeable to hospital policies
- Presence of consultant support of diabetes mellitus (DM) team.
- No severe hypoglycemia
- No medication interference
- Tolerating per os (PO) nutrition
- No concern for insulin pump/CGM malfunction
- No ionizing/magnetic radiation exposure.

Box 11
Contraindications to insulin pump/continuous glucose monitor systems[28,56,62]

- Impaired level of consciousness (except during short-term anesthesia)
- Inability to correctly demonstrate appropriate system settings
- Critical illness requiring intensive care
- Psychiatric illness that interferes with self-management abilities
- DKA and hyperosmolar hyperglycemic state
- Refusal or unwillingness to participate in self-care
- Lack of system supplies
- Lack of trained health care providers, diabetes educators, or diabetes specialists
- Patient at risk for suicide

Box 12
Patient responsibilities[53,56]

- Sign a patient agreement
- Agrees to notify health care provider (HCP) if observing glucose excursions
- Understand trend arrows and notify HCP if noted
- Bring sufficient supplies
- Maintain their own device
- Change their sites as directed
- Device supplies storage per policy and returned upon discharge

Box 13
Health care provider responsibilities[53,56]

- Review policy and obtain agreement
- Document technology certification program completion
- Understand alarms
- Use of vendor training programs through websites
- Understand interstitial fluid (ISF) lags capillary glucose when recognizing/treating hypoglycemia
- Document medication supplements that might interfere with CGM
- Ensure off-label use is consistent with medical practice with appropriate precautions
- Regular reviews for continued ability to safety operate devices and change sites
- Inspect sites/location every shift
- Remove and safely store devices for radiological procedures
- Review for orders for insulin coverage during time pump is removed
- Technology support availability
- Check POC BGs per policy
- Document boluses, modes, nursing logs, and patient logs
- Recommend alternate care if patient ability changes
- Education with alternate discharge dosage if there are changes

Box 14
Establishing an insulin pump/continuous glucose monitor system/ hospital system responsibilities[38,39,53,54,56,65]

- Develop protocols with diabetes care specialist
- Establish goals based on American Diabetes Association (ADA) Standards of Care 2024.
- Require patient to bring sufficient supplies
- Develop protocols for elective procedures and surgeries
- Switch AID Systems from "auto" to "manual" mode when admitted
- Predefine assignments with clear structure surrounding monitoring/interpretation of data

- Develop appropriate security protocols, dedicated data storage, visualization tools, and adequate cyber insurance coverage (also known as "data at rest")
- Integrate data into electronic health record (EHR) to have access to information
- Determine number of laboratory or POC BG needed while on devices
- Develop unique identifier to track devices in EHR
- Identify CGM data in EHR to distinguish from laboratory glucose results
- Develop criteria to identify data that need interventions
- Arrange CGM results to be automatically uploaded to EHR
- Manage CGM data with same safety/security measures for all Personal Health Information (PHI)
- Develop policies for use of systems in atypical scenarios
- Provide interpretation services to translate patient agreements
- State in policy that treatment decisions will be based on hospital-calibrated readings
- Storage of agreements in EHR
- Develop policies when to suspend/discontinue systems
- Survey the HCP for system outcome improvements
- HCP use of "follow" features of CGM on a unit dedicated device
- Use of CGM online vendor platforms data transfers

Box 15
Various causes of hyperglycemia in insulin pump wearers[66–70]

Infusion set issues:
- Kinked, dislodged, leaking, clogged, or tubing or cannula
- Air bubbles in tubing especially when drawing up cold insulin
- Prolonged disconnection (sports, sexual intimacy, swimming/bathing)

Pump-related issues:
- Batteries died
- No insulin or bad insulin
- Pump failure
- Incorrect pump settings
- Underbolused or no bolus dose

Skin-Related issues
- Insulin malabsorption
- Infection at site

Metabolic issues
- Menstrual cycle
- Infection, illness, injury
- New medications, especially steroids
- Recent hypoglycemia
- Change in eating patterns or food
- Stress
- Decreased physical activity
- Change in sleeping cycles

Other issues
- Glucometer errors/strip issues

Box 14 discusses how to establish an insulin pump/CGM system along with hospital system responsibilities.

TROUBLESHOOTING/HYPERGLYCEMIA PROTOCOL/WHEN TO DISCONNECT PUMP

Persons with diabetes and their family and HCP must be on guard for potential causes of both hypoglycemia and hyperglycemia. **Box 15** discusses the various causes of hyperglycemia in insulin pump wearers.

SUMMARY

Many hospital systems have developed policy, procedures, and patient agreement forms. The Continuous Glucose Monitors and Automated Insulin Dosing System in the Hospital Consensus Guidelines have a sample patient agreement in their guidelines.[56] Other algorithms and pathways obtained from the literature can be helpful to allow hospital systems to develop their own.[28,57]

CLINICS CARE POINTS

- Research trials established intensive insulin management utilizing either MDI or use of an insulin pump achieving lower hemoglobin A1C.
- Estimated 350,000 persons wear an insulin pump and 2.4 million wear a CGM in the United States.
- Many diabetes organizations have generated position statements to allow the most optimal diabetes treatment, even when hospitalized.
- The Diabetes Technology Society Hospital Consensus Guideline Panel developed 77 recommendations to support hospitalized patients with diabetes and met again in 2023 to review progress.

DISCLOSURE

The author was a certified Medtronic insulin pump and sensor trainer in the past but has not trained patients in more than 5 years.

REFERENCES

1. International Diabetes Federation, Diabetes Atlas, 10th edition, Available at: https://diabetesatlas.org/atlas/tenth-edition/ (Accessed 25 May 2024).
2. American Diabetes Association, Statistics about diabetes, Available at: https://diabetes.org/about-diabetes/statistics/about-diabetes (Accessed 25 May 2024).
3. Centers for Disease Control and Prevention, National Diabetes Statistics Report 2024, Available at: https://www.cdc.gov/diabetes/php/data-research/?CDC_AAref_Val=https://www.cdc.gov/diabetes/data/statistics-report/index.html (Accessed 28 August 2024).
4. Mulvey A., More people being diagnosed with type 1 diabetes. Juvenile diabetes research Foundation blog. 2020, Available at: https://www.jdrf.org/blog/2020/02/18/more-people-being-diagnosed-type-1-diabetes/ (Accessed 24 May 2024).
5. Nguyen S, Davis GM, Vasudevan MM. Clinical practice update: inpatient insulin pump and integrated insulin delivery systems. Diabetes management in hospitalized patients: a comprehensive clinical guide. Springer; 2024. p. 95–116.

6. Didyuk O, Econom N, Guardia A, et al. Continuous glucose monitoring devices: past, present, and future focus on the history and evolution of technological innovation. J Diabetes Sci Technol 2021;15(3):676–83.

7. Diabetes Control and Complications Trial Research Group. The effect of intensive treatment of diabetes on the development and progression of long-term complications in insulin-dependent diabetes mellitus. N Engl J Med 1993;329(14): 977–86.

8. Epidemiology of diabetes interventions complications research group. Epidemiology of diabetes interventions and complications (EDIC): design, implementation, and preliminary results of a long-term follow-up of the diabetes control and complications trial cohort. Diabetes Care 1999;22(1):99.

9. Shepard E., Diabetes technology: the future is today, UAB expert says, Available at: https://www.uab.edu/reporter/patient-care/advances/item/10135-diabetes-technology-the-future-is-today#:~:text~The%20Centers%20for%20Disease%20Control,are%20using%20CGMs%2C%20Basu%20says, 2023 (Accessed 25 May 2024).

10. McAdams BH, Rizvi AA. An overview of insulin pumps and glucose sensors for the generalist. J Clin Med 2016;5(1):5.

11. NA. Insulin pump adoption seen climbing 21% in 2021 on wearables boom: survey. Medtechdive blog. March 5, 2021. Available at: https://www.medtechdive.com/news/insulin-pump-adoption-seen-climbing-21-in-2021-on-wearables-boom-survey/596207/.

12. Bode BW, Sabbah HT, Gross TM, et al. Diabetes management in the new millennium using insulin pump therapy. Diabetes/metabolism research and reviews 2002;18(S1):S14–20.

13. Kesavadev J, Saboo B, Krishna MB, et al. Evolution of insulin delivery devices: from syringes, pens, and pumps to DIY artificial pancreas. Diabetes Ther 2020; 11(6):1251–69.

14. Penfornis A, Personeni E, Borot S. Evolution of devices in diabetes management. Diabetes Technol Ther 2011;13(S1). S-93-S-102.

15. Alsaleh FM, Smith FJ, Keady S, et al. Insulin pumps: from inception to the present and toward the future. J Clin Pharm Ther 2010;35(2):127–38.

16. Sims EK, Carr AL, Oram RA, et al. 100 years of insulin: celebrating the past, present and future of diabetes therapy. Nature medicine 2021;27(7):1154–64.

17. Reece SW, Williams CLH. Insulin pump class: back to the basics of pump therapy. Diabetes Spectr 2014;27(2):135.

18. American Association of Diabetes Educators. Continuous subcutaneous insulin infusion (CSII) without and with sensor integration. Association of Diabetes Care & Education Specialists; 2018.

19. American Diabetes Association. The history of a wonderful thing we call insulin 5/25/2024. Available at: https://diabetes.org/blog/history-wonderful-thing-we-call-insulin.

20. Hirsch IB, Juneja R, Beals JM, et al. The evolution of insulin and how it informs therapy and treatment choices. Endocr Rev 2020;41(5):733–55.

21. American Diabetes Association. Insulin pumps consumer guide. Available at: https://consumerguide.diabetes.org/collections/pumps. Accessed May 24, 2024.

22. Valla V. Therapeutics of diabetes mellitus: focus on insulin analogues and insulin pumps. J Diabetes Res 2010;2010:178372.

23. American Diabetes Association. Consumer guide: insulin. Available at: https://consumerguide.diabetes.org/collections/insulin. Accessed May 25, 2024.

24. Clarke SF, Foster JR. A history of blood glucose meters and their role in self-monitoring of diabetes mellitus. Br J Biomed Sci 2012;69(2):83–93.

25. Garg SK. Past, present, and future of continuous glucose monitors. Diabetes Technol Ther 2023;25(S3). S-1-S-4.

26. Kumareswaran K, Evans ML, Hovorka R. Artificial pancreas: an emerging approach to treat type 1 diabetes. Expet Rev Med Dev 2009;6(4):401–10.

27. Medtronic. Innovation Milestones- innovating since 1983. Available at: https://www.medtronicdiabetes.com/about-medtronic-innovation/milestone-timeline. Accessed May 27, 2024.

28. Umpierrez GE, Klonoff DC. Diabetes technology update: use of insulin pumps and continuous glucose monitoring in the hospital. Diabetes Care 2018;41(8):1579–89.

29. Bochicchio GV, Nasraway S, Moore L, et al. Results of a multicenter prospective pivotal trial of the first inline continuous glucose monitor in critically ill patients. J Trauma Acute Care Surg 2017;82(6):1049–54.

30. Faulkner S. OptiScan raises $20m for bedside glucose monitoring system. Drug Delivery Business News. 2024. Available at: https://www.drugdeliverybusiness.com/optiscan-raises-20m-for-bedside-glucose-monitoring-system/.

31. Whooley S. 7 Medtech Advances to Improve Diabetes Treatment. Massdevice Medical Network. Available at: https://www.massdevice.com/7-medtech-advances-that-can-improve-diabetes-treatment/ (Accessed 25 May 2024).

32. The diaTRIBE Foundation. Continous glucose monitors. Available at: https://diatribe.org/diabetes-technology/continuous-glucose-monitors. Accessed June 2, 2024.

33. American Diabetes Assocation. Consumer guide: CGM. Available at: https://consumerguide.diabetes.org/collections/cgm. Accessed June 24, 2024.

34. Association of diabetes care and education specialist. Find & Compare insulin pumps. Available at: https://www.adces.org/danatech/insulin-pumps/find-and-compare-insulin-pumps. Accessed June 2, 2024.

35. American Diabetes Assocation. 7. Diabetes technology: standards of care in diabetes—2024. Diabetes Care 2024;47(Supplement_1):S126–44.

36. Medtronic. Sensor glucose vs blood glucose: why sensor glucose does not equal blood glucose 5/27/2024. Available at: https://www.medtronicdiabetes.com/customer-support/sensors-and-transmitters-support/why-sensor-glucose-does-not-equal-blood-glucose.

37. Davis GM, Galindo RJ, Migdal AL, et al. Diabetes technology in the inpatient setting for management of hyperglycemia. Endocrinol Metabol Clin 2020;49(1):79–93.

38. The Association of Diabetes Care & Education Specialist. The role of the diabetes care and education specialist in the hospital setting. Sci Diabetes Self Manag Care 2022;48(3):184–91. https://doi.org/10.1177/26350106221094332.

39. Tian T, Aaron RE, Yeung AM, et al. Use of continuous glucose monitors in the hospital: the Diabetes Technology Society hospital meeting report 2023. J Diabetes Sci Technol 2023;17(5):1392–418.

40. Templer S. Closed-loop insulin delivery systems: past, present, and future directions. Front Endocrinol 2022;13:919942.

41. Sherr JL, Heinemann L, Fleming GA, et al. Automated insulin delivery: benefits, challenges, and recommendations. A consensus report of the Joint diabetes technology working group of the European Association for the study of diabetes and the American diabetes Association. Diabetes Care 2022;45(12):3058–74.

42. Burnside MJ, Lewis DM, Crocket HR, et al. Open-source automated insulin delivery in type 1 diabetes. N Engl J Med 2022;387(10):869–81. https://doi.org/10.1056/NEJMoa2203913.

43. ADCES Professional Practice Committee, CGM & pump integration: rapid data collection using CGM integrated with insulin pumps, Available at: https://www.adces.org/danatech/insulin-pumps/training-clients-patients/cgm-pump-integration, 2024 (Accessed 6 June 2024).

44. Lewis D. History and Perspective on DIY closed looping. J Diabetes Sci Technol 2019;13(4):790–3.

45. Sherr J, Tamborlane WV. Past, present, and future of insulin pump therapy: a better shot at diabetes control. Mount Sinai J Med 2008;75(4):352–61.

46. Bergenstal RM, Tamborlane WV, Ahmann A, et al. Effectiveness of sensor-augmented insulin-pump therapy in type 1 diabetes. N Engl J Med 2010;363(4):311–20.

47. Juvenile Diabetes Research Foundation Continuous Glucose Monitoring Study Group. Continuous glucose monitoring and intensive treatment of type 1 diabetes. N Engl J Med 2008;359(14):1464–76.

48. Maahs DM, Calhoun P, Buckingham BA, et al. A randomized trial of a home system to reduce nocturnal hypoglycemia in type 1 diabetes. Diabetes Care 2014;37(7):1885–91.

49. Buckingham BA, Raghinaru D, Cameron F, et al. Predictive low-glucose insulin suspension reduces duration of nocturnal hypoglycemia in children without increasing Ketosis. Diabetes Care 2015;38(7):1197–204.

50. Forlenza GP, Li Z, Buckingham BA, et al. Predictive low-glucose suspend reduces hypoglycemia in adults, adolescents, and children with type 1 diabetes in an at-home randomized crossover study: results of the PROLOG trial. Diabetes Care 2018;41(10):2155–61.

51. Abraham MB, Nicholas JA, Smith GJ, et al. Reduction in hypoglycemia with the predictive low-glucose management system: a long-term randomized controlled trial in adolescents with type 1 diabetes. Diabetes Care 2018;41(2):303–10.

52. American Diabetes Association. 16. Diabetes care in the hospital: standards of care in diabetes—2024. Diabetes Care 2024;47(Supplement_1):S295–306.

53. Perez-Guzman MC, Shang T, Zhang JY, et al. Continuous monitoring in the hospital. Endocrinol Metab (Seoul) 2021;36(2):240–55.

54. Galindo RJ, Aleppo G, Klonoff DC, et al. Implementation of continuous glucose monitoring in the hospital: emergent considerations for remote glucose monitoring during the COVID-19 pandemic. J Diabetes Sci Technol 2020;14(4):822–32.

55. Joint Commission. Quick Safety 59: Safe patient use of insulin pumps and CGM devices during hospitalization. 2021.

56. Galindo RJ, Umpierrez GE, Rushakoff RJ, et al. Continuous glucose monitors and automated insulin dosing systems in the hospital consensus guideline. J Diabetes Sci Technol 2020;14(6):1035–64.

57. Rotruck S, Suszan L, Vigersky R, et al. Should continuous subcutaneous insulin infusion (CSII) pumps be used during the perioperative period? Development of a clinical decision algorithm. AANA J 2018;86(3):194–200.

58. Perez-Guzman MC, Duggan E, Gibanica S, et al. Continuous glucose monitoring in the operating room and cardiac intensive care unit. Diabetes Care 2021;44(3):e50–2.

59. Duggan E, Chen Y. Glycemic management in the operating room: screening, monitoring, oral hypoglycemics, and insulin therapy. Curr Diabetes Rep 2019; 19(11):134.
60. Feig DS, Donovan LE, Corcoy R, et al. Continuous glucose monitoring in pregnant women with type 1 diabetes (CONCEPTT): a multicentre international randomised controlled trial. Lancet 2017;390(10110):2347–59.
61. Polsky S, Garcetti R. CGM, pregnancy, and remote monitoring. Diabetes Technol Ther 2017;19(S3). S-49-S-59.
62. Yeh T, Yeung M, Mendelsohn Curanaj FA. Managing patients with insulin pumps and continuous glucose monitors in the hospital: to wear or not to wear. Curr Diabetes Rep 2021;21:1–11.
63. Korytkowski MT, Muniyappa R, Antinori-Lent K, et al. Management of hyperglycemia in hospitalized adult patients in non-critical care settings: an Endocrine Society clinical practice guideline. J Clin Endocrinol Metab 2022;107(8):2101–28.
64. Nguyen S, Davis GM, Vasudevan MM. Clinical practice update: inpatient insulin pump and integrated insulin delivery systems. In: Schulman-Rosenbaum RC, editor. Diabetes management in hospitalized patients: a comprehensive clinical guide. Springer International Publishing; 2023. p. 95–116.
65. Ribeiro Júnior MAF, Brenner M, Nguyen ATM, et al. Resuscitative endovascular balloon occlusion of the aorta (REBOA): an updated review. Rev Col Bras Cir 2018;45:e1709.
66. Diabetes.co.UK.: the global diabetes community. Insulin pumps. May 14, 2017. Available at: http://www.diabetes.co.uk/insulin/Insulin-pumps.html. Accessed May 8, 2017.
67. Walsh J, Roberts R. Pumping insulin: everything for success on an insulin pump and CGM. 6th edition. Torrey Pines Press; 2017.
68. Wolpert H. Smart Pumping for people with diabetes. A practical approach to mastering the insulin pump. American Diabetes Association; 2002.
69. Insulin, infusion set troubleshooting guide, Available at: https://www.adces.org/docs/default-source/handouts/insulinrelated/handout_hcp_ir_troubleshootingguide.pdf?Status=Master&sfvrsn=4b346359_19 (Accessed 28 August 2024).
70. McCrea DL. A primer on insulin pump therapy for health care providers. Nurs Clin North Am 2017;52(4):553–64.

Managing Heart Disease in Persons with Diabetes

Deborah L. McCrea, EdD, MSN, RN, FNP-BC, CNS, CNE, CEN, CFRN, EMT-P

KEYWORDS

- Type 1 diabetes • Type 2 diabetes • Prediabetes • Gestational diabetes
- Cardiovascular complications • Diabetes control and complications trial (DCCT)
- Epidemiology of diabetes interventions and complications (EDIC)

KEY POINTS

- There are an estimated 38 million persons in the United States who have diabetes mellitus, both diagnosed and undiagnosed.
- Cardiovascular (CV) disease is a common complication in persons with diabetes (PWD).
- CV diseases including cardiac, cerebrovascular, and peripheral vascular diseases and are the leading causes of death in PWD.
- Complications include ischemic heart disease, peripheral artery disease, heart failure, and stroke.
- Several diabetes and CV professional organizations publish yearly standards of care based on global evidence-based research in diabetes and CV health.

INTRODUCTION

Currently, it is estimated that almost 38 million persons in the United States have diabetes mellitus (DM), both diagnosed and undiagnosed. Approximately 352,000 people younger than 20 years old have diabetes with 304,000 who have type 1 diabetes (T1D).[1] Diabetes is classified into several categories including T1D, type 2 diabetes (T2D), gestational DM, and other types related to genetic causes, exocrine pancreatic disorders, and medication-induced diabetes.[2] **Box 1** discusses the categories of DM.

General Diabetes Complications

One of the highest causes of complications in persons with diabetes (PWD) is cardiovascular (CV)-related issues.

Complications, in general, are due to insulin deficiency or insulin resistance, with persistent hyperglycemia, dyslipidemia, and other metabolic pathways disorders. In

Department of Graduate Studies, UTHealth Houston, Cizik School of Nursing, 6901 Bertner, Suite 695, Houston, TX 77030, USA
E-mail address: Deborah.L.McCrea@uth.tmc.edu

Crit Care Nurs Clin N Am 37 (2025) 53–66
https://doi.org/10.1016/j.cnc.2024.10.001 ccnursing.theclinics.com

---

Box 1
Categories of Diabetes

Type 1 diabetes
- Is due to autoimmune β-cell destruction, usually leading to absolute insulin deficiency, including latent autoimmune diabetes in adults

Type 2 diabetes
- Is due to a nonautoimmune progressive loss of adequate β-cell insulin secretion, frequently on the background of insulin resistance and metabolic syndrome

Gestational diabetes mellitus (DM)
- Is DM diagnosed in the second or third trimester of pregnancy that was not clearly overt DM prior to gestation or other types of DM occurring throughout pregnancy, such as type 1 diabetes

Other types of diabetes due to other causes
- Monogenic diabetes syndromes such as neonatal diabetes and maturity-onset diabetes of the young
- Diseases of the exocrine pancreas including cystic fibrosis and pancreatitis
- Drug or chemical-induced diabetes including glucocorticoid use, in treatment of people with HIV, or after organ transplantation

Data from American Diabetes Association. 2. Diagnosis and classification of diabetes: Standards of care in diabetes—2024. Diabetes Care. 2024;47(Supplement_1):S20-S42.

---

the past, DM complications were divided into microvascular issues including retinopathy, neuropathy, and nephropathy and macrovascular complications such as CV, cerebrovascular, and peripheral vascular diseases. Researchers are finding an interplay of various risk factors such as glucose free fatty acids, oxidants, inflammatory stress proteins, advanced glycation end product (AGE), vasotropic hormones, thrombotic factors and vasoconstrictors along with protective factors such as hormones, cytokines, antioxidants, anti-inflammatory factors, anti-AGE, activated protein C, and vasodilators. Because of these new discoveries, experts are now recategorizing DM complications based on either vascular, parenchymal, and hybrid (vascular and

---

Table 1
Pathologic categories of diabetes complications

Vascular Tissues	Parenchymal Tissues	Hybrid (Vascular-Parenchymal Mixed)
Vascular complications are predominantly cardiovascular or vascular tissues, such as the arteries. • Renal glomeruli • Myocardium • Central nervous system vasculature • Central nervous system (strokes)	Parenchymal tissue complications affecting nonvascular organ components. • Malignancies • Alzheimer's disease • Osteoarthritide in bone and cartilage structure issues (including decreased bone remodeling, increased synovial inflammation, promotion of chondrocyte apoptosis, and altered extracellular matrix structure in bone/cartilage) • Periodontitis • Poor wound healing	Diverse pathologies of organs, mainly caused by metabolic changes induced by insulin deficiency, insulin resistance, or both. • Retinopathy • Neuropathy • Poor wound healing

Data from Yu MG, Gordin D, Fu J, Park K, Li Q, King GL. Protective factors and the pathogenesis of complications in diabetes. Endocrine Reviews. 2023;45(2):227-252. doi:10.1210/endrev/bnad030

parenchymal-mixed) origins. See **Table 1** to view the pathologic categories of DM complications.[3]

Diabetes and Cardiovascular Complications in Persons with Type 1 and Type 2 Diabetes

Cardiovascular disease (CVD), including cardiac, cerebrovascular, and peripheral vascular diseases, are the leading causes of death among PWD and have a 2 to 8 times greater risk of CVD.[4–7] Complications from ischemic heart disease, peripheral artery disease, heart failure (HF), and stroke can result in 50% increased mortality in persons with T2D.[8] Approximately half of the deaths of individuals with DM are attributable to CVD. Individuals with T2D have a twofold increased risk of CV mortality compared with healthy individuals. PWD often have other conditions coexisting including hypertension and dyslipidemia along with the DM condition itself that causes an exacerbation of this condition. HF also is another major cause of morbidity and mortality including a twofold increase in HF hospitalizations.[4,5]

In persons with T1D, data from 2 groundbreaking research studies reviewing the efficacy of intensive glycemic control, known as the Diabetes Control and Complications Trial (DCCT) and the Epidemiology of Diabetes Interventions and Complications (EDIC) study confirmed the reduction of several DM-related complications with intensive insulin therapy. The DCCT study found people who were on intensive insulin therapy with either multiple daily insulin injections or the use of an insulin pump had a 76% reduction in retinopathy, 56% reduction in nephropathy, and 60% reduction in neuropathy. Some of these same participants were then enrolled in the EDIC study to assess CVD reduction and found CVD events decreased by 42%, nonfatal myocardial infarctions (MIs), stroke, or death from CVD was reduced by 57%.[9,10] Current research has found that T1D is associated with almost a 3-fold to 10-fold increase in mortality rates compared with the general population.[11]

Prediabetes

It is also estimated that almost 100,000 million persons have prediabetes, which is defined as impaired fasting glucose of 100 to 125 mg/dL, or Hbg1Ac of 5.7% to 6.4% or impaired glucose tolerance where a 2-h plasma glucose level after administration of a 75-g oral glucose tolerance test yields a plasma glucose level of 140 to 199 mg/dL. Up to 70% of individuals with prediabetes will eventually develop DM. Prediabetes is associated with an increased risk of CV disease and all-cause mortality even though they have not been diagnosed with DM yet.[2,12,13]

There is evidence that prediabetes is a "toxic state" and associated with pathophysiological changes in several tissues and organs including the CV system due to atherosclerotic changes in the vessels. Metabolic syndrome often coexisting with increased fibrinogen and high-sensitivity C-reactive peptide puts them at higher risk for atheroma development. The conditions of hyperglycemia, insulin resistance, inflammation, and other metabolic dysfunctions cause endothelial vasodilation and fibrinolytic changes leading to these chronic complications and risk of coronary artery disease (CAD), diastolic HF, chronic renal disease, ophthalmologic issues, neurologic concerns, gastrointestinal issues, and various cancers.[14–16]

A meta-analysis of 129 studies reviewed data involving over 10 million people to assess for an association between prediabetes and risk of all-cause mortality and CV disease. They concluded prediabetes was associated with an increased risk of mortality from CV disease.[17] **Box 2** describes the criteria for screening for DM and prediabetes in asymptomatic adults.

Box 2
Criteria for screening for diabetes mellitus and prediabetes in asymptomatic adults

Testing should be considered in adults with overweight or obesity (body mass index $\geq$ 25 kg/m^2 or $\geq$23 kg/m^2 in Asian American individuals) who have one or more of the following risk factors:
- First-degree relative with diabetes mellitus (DM) high-risk race and ethnicity (eg, African American, Latino, Native American, Asian American, Pacific Islander)
- History of cardiovascular disease
- Hypertension ($\geq$130/80 mm Hg or on therapy for hypertension)
- High-density lipoprotein (HDL) cholesterol level 250 mg/dL (>2.8 mmol/L)
- Individuals with polycystic ovary syndrome
- Physical inactivity
- Other clinical conditions associated with insulin resistance (eg, severe obesity, acanthosis nigricans)

People with prediabetes (hemoglobin A1c (A1c) $\geq$ 5.7%, impaired fasting glucose, or impaired glucose tolerate should be tested yearly.

People who were diagnosed with gestational diabetes (GDM) should have lifelong testing at least every 3 years. For all other people, testing for diabetes should begin at the age of 35 years.

If results are normal, repeat in minimum of 3-year intervals, with more frequent testing depending on initial results/risk status.

People with HIV, exposure to high-risk medicines, history of pancreatitis

Data from American Diabetes Association. 2. Diagnosis and classification of diabetes: Standards of care in diabetes—2024. Diabetes Care. 2024;47(Supplement_1):S20-S42.

Diabetes-related complications include many risk factors in PWD. **Table 2** discusses CV risk factors associated with DM-related complications in persons 18 years and older.[1]

Management of Cardiovascular Risk Factors

The following will discuss evidence-based comprehensive management of CV risk factors for persons with T2D. These data are generated from scientific papers and yearly standards of care guidelines from esteem organizations such as the American Heart Association (AHA) and the American Diabetes Association (ADA). This information will review updates to lifestyle modifications, oral agents that have cardioprotective properties, hypertension reduction, hyperlipidemia control, thrombus preventions, and updated CV testing guidelines.

Previously, guideline protocols and scientific position statements did not have sufficient evidence that glucose lowering medications would reduce CV events. However, after more research, the AHA found that newer antihyperglycemic agents have been found to have CV safety and subsequent reduction in CV death, MI, stroke, and HF. CV deaths have decreased in the United States for persons with and without DM; however, it is still quite high. These guidelines can also be utilized for appropriateness for those with T1D and prediabetes as the AHA statement did not address these categories specifically. **Box 3** will discuss lifestyle management guidelines for the reduction of CV risk factor reduction.[18]

Box 4 will discuss obesity and weight loss management guidelines for CV risk factor reduction[18,19]

Box 5 will discuss antihyperglycemic agents that have some CV risk reduction. **Table 3** will discuss blood pressure management for CV risk reduction.[20]

Table 2
Percentages of factors associated with diabetes mellitus-related complications in persons ≥18 years old who have diabetes mellitus

Risk Factors for DM-Related Complications	Percentages (95% CI)
Smoking	
• Current tobacco use	• 22.1 (18.7–26.0)
• Current cigarette smoker	• 14.6 (12.2–17.3)
• Former cigarette smoker	• 36.0 (30.5–41.8)
Overweight and obesity, according to body mass index (BMI)	
• BMI ≥ 25.0 kg/m^2	• 89.8 (87.2–92.0)
• BMI 25.0–29.9 kg/m^2	• 26.9 (24.0–30.0)
• BMI 30.0–39.9 kg/m^2	• 47.1 (43.3–51.0)
• BMI ≥ 40.0 kg/m^2	• 15.7 (12.4–19.7)
A1c	
• A1c ≥ 7.0%	• 47.4 (41.1–53.8)
• A1c 7.0–7.9%	• 22.9 (18.7–27.8
• A1c 8.0–9.0%	• 11.5 (8.3–15.7)
• A1c > 9.0%	• 13.0 (10.5–15.9)
High blood pressure	
• Blood pressure ≥ 130/80 mmHg or taking antihypertensive medication	• 80.6 (77.5–83.3)
• Blood pressure ≥ 140/90 mmHg or taking antihypertensive medication	• 70.8 (66.8–74.5)
High cholesterol, according to non-HDL cholesterol	
• Non-HDL ≥130 mg/dL	• 39.5 (33.1–46.2)
• Non-HDL 130–159 mg/dL	• 19.9 (16.3–24.1)
• Non-HDL 160–189 mg/dL	• 11.5 (8.1–16.1)
• Non-HDL ≥190 mg/dL	• 8.0 (5.7–11.1)

Abbreviations: DM, diabetes mellitus; HDL, high-density lipoprotein; 95% CI, 95% confidence interval.
Data from Centers for Disease Control and Prevention. National Diabetes Statistics Report. 2024, January 8.

Box 3
Lifestyle management guidelines for reduction of cardiovascular risk factor reduction

- Diabetes self-management education and support
- Medical nutrition therapy tailored by a dietician team including approximately 1200 to 1800 kcal/day, intake of various macro/micronutrients, sodium awareness, carbohydrate reduction, fat intake to less than 30%, and protein to above 15%, periodic meal replacements, addressing food insecurity issues, setting up eating patterns/meal planning, intermittent fasting, and religious fasting.
- Physical activity of approximately 175 minutes/week of moderate intensity aerobic activity, resistance training or both
- Smoking cessation
- Psychosocial care including assessment for diabetes mellitus distress, anxiety, depression, eating disorders, serious mental illness, cognitive capacity/impairment, and sleep health

- Alcohol: needs further research because some studies found light to moderate intake benefitted A1c, lipids, and myocardial infarction reduction whereas heavier alcohol consumption was associated with higher risk which may be due to an increase in blood pressure and high-density lipoprotein levels.

Data from Joseph JJ, Deedwania P, Acharya T, et al. Comprehensive management of cardiovascular risk factors for adults with type 2 diabetes: a scientific statement from the American Heart Association. Circulation. 2022;145(9):e722-e759; American Diabetes Association. 5. Facilitating Positive Health Behaviors and Well-being to Improve Health Outcomes: Standards of Care in Diabetes—2024. Diabetes Care. 2023;47(Supplement_1):S77-S110. doi:10.2337/dc24-S005

Box 4

Obesity and weight loss management guidelines for cardiovascular risk factor reduction

Pharmacologic therapy adjuncts to diet, physical activity, and behavioral therapy
*Found to have cardiovascular (CV) safety and additional benefit of lowering A1c.
- Orlistat
- Lorcaserin
- Liraglutide
- Naltrexone/bupropion
- Phentermine/topiramate
- Liraglutide at lower doses among those with atherosclerotic cardiovascular disease (ASCVD) or high CV risk
- Nonweight loss-approved medications commonly used in type 2 diabetes (T2D) lower weight, including pramlintide, sodium-glucose co-transporter-2 inhibitors (SGLT-2I), metformin, and other glucagon-like peptide-1 receptor agonists (GLP-1RAs)
- The STEP (Semaglutide Treatment Effect in People with Obesity) study demonstrated tremendous impact of GLP-1RA treatment with semaglutide on weight loss and CV risk factors

Surgical interventions
- Metabolic surgery is recommended to treat persons who have T2D with body mass index (BMI) $\geq$ 40 kg/m^2 and in those with BMI 35.0 to 39.9 kg/m^2 without durable weight loss and improvement in comorbidities with nonsurgical methods and should be considered in those with T2D and BMI of 30.0 to 34.9 kg/m^2 without similar improvements.

Data from Joseph JJ, Deedwania P, Acharya T, et al. Comprehensive management of cardiovascular risk factors for adults with type 2 diabetes: A scientific statement from the American Heart Association. Circulation. 2022;145(9):e722-e759; American Diabetes Association. 5. Facilitating positive health behaviors and well-being to improve health outcomes: Standards of care in diabetes—2024. Diabetes Care. 2023;47(Supplement_1):S77-S110. https://doi.org/10.2337/dc24-S005.

Box 5

Antihyperglycemic agents for cardiovascular risk reduction

Dipeptidyl Peptidate-4 Inhibitors (DPP-4)
- Saxagliptin
- Alogliptin
- Sitagliptin
- Linagliptin

DPP-4 inhibitors reduced A1c by 0.2% to 0.36% but showed no reduction in major adverse cardiovascular events (MACEs). There are concerns for increasing the risk of heart failure (HF) with saxagliptin but not the other DPP-4 inhibitors

Glucagon-Like Peptide-1 Receptor Agonist (GLP-1RA)
  This category of medications has potential indirect CV effects including increased insulin secretion, decreased glucagon release, increased natriuresis, decreased blood volume, decreased appetite, decreased body weight, decreased inflammation, increased glucose utilization, decreased fatty acid utilization, increased coronary flow, and increased heart rate

- Liraglutide
- Lixisenatide
- Albiglutide
- Dulaglutide
- Efpeglenatide
- Exenatide
- Semaglutide

Lixisenatide, exenatide, and oral semaglutide were noninferior to standard care, liraglutide, semaglutide SQ, albiglutide, dulaglutide, and efpeglenatide showed a statistically significant 12% to 27% MACE reduction.

This reduction was driven by fewer CV deaths with liraglutide, less myocardial infarction (MI) with albiglutide, and fewer strokes with injectable semaglutide and dulaglutide.

GLP-1RAs reduced risk of 3-point MACE (10%–12%), CV mortality (12%–13%), all-cause mortality (12%), MI (6%–9%), and stroke (13%–14%).

There was no significant effect on hospitalizations for HF (HHF). GLP-1RAs performed better among individuals without HF, except for albiglutide.

Sodium-Glucose Cotransporter-2 Inhibitors (SGLT-2I)
- Empagliflozin
- Canagliflozin
- Dapagliflozin
- Ertugliflozin
- Sotagliflozin

SGLT-2Is lowered A1c (0.36%–0.58%), systolic blood pressure (SBP) (2–3.9 mm Hg), and weight (1.0–2.8 kg) compared with placebo over 1 to 4 years.

The SGLT-2I trials have shown a congruently lower risk (27%–35%) of HHF.

Meta-analyses of cardiovascular outcome trail (excluding ertugliflozin and sotagliflozin) reveal that SGLT-2Is reduced MACE (11%), CV mortality or HHF (23%), all-cause mortality (15%), MI (11%), and CV mortality (16%) with no effect on stroke

Real-world observational studies have largely shown similar findings with reduced HHF and CV mortality, but additionally suggest lower risk of MI and stroke.

FDA Regulatory Approval
The FDA has been approved the following SGT-2I with the following labels:
CV death reduction:
- Empagliflozin

MACE reduction:
- Liraglutide
- Semaglutide (subcutaneous)
- Canagliflozin in adults with type 2 diabetes (T2D) and established cardiovascular disease (CVD)
- Dulaglutide in adults with T2D and established CVD or multiple CVD risk factors

Decrease in HHF in T2D and established CVD or multiple CVD risk factors and a decrease HHF and CVD-related death in HF and reduced ejection fraction, with or without diabetes mellitus (DM):
- Dapagliflozin

Other treatment recommendations per the American Diabetes Association[5]
T2D with established:
- ASCVD/kidney disease: start with an SGLT-2I or GLP-1RA with demonstrated CV benefit
- ASCVD/multiple ASCVD risk factors/kidney disease: start with an SGLT-2I with demonstrated CV benefit to reduce major adverse CV events and/or HF
- ASCVD/multiple ASCVD risk factors: start with GLP-1RA with demonstrated CV benefit to reduce risk of major adverse CV events
- ASCVD or multiple risk factors for ASCVD: start combined therapy with SGLT-2I with demonstrated CV benefit + GLP-1RA with demonstrated CV benefit may be an additive reduction of risk of adverse CV and kidney events
- Heart failure (HF) with preserved/reduced ejection fraction: start with SGLT-2I (including SGLT1/2 inhibitor) with proven benefit to reduce risk of worsening HF and CV death
- HF with either preserved or reduced ejection fraction: start with SGLT-2I with proven benefit to improve symptoms, physical limitations, and quality of life

- Chronic kidney disease with albuminuria treated with maximum tolerated doses of angiotensin-converting enzyme-inhibitor (ACEi) or angiotensin receptor blocker (ARB): add finerenone to improve CV outcomes and reduce risk of CKD progression
- Asymptomatic stage B HF or with high risk of or established CV disease: start with SGLT-2I (including SGLT-2 or SGLT1/2 inhibitors) to reduce risk of hospitalization
- Kidney disease: finerenone is recommended to reduce the risk of hospitalization for HF.
- Stable HF: metformin may be continued for glucose lowering if estimated glomerular filtration rate remains greater than 30 mL/min/1.73 m^2 but should be avoided in unstable or hospitalized individuals with HF

All Persons with Diabetes with established:
- ASCVD or aged $\geq$55 years with additional CV risk factors: add ACEi or ARB therapy to reduce risk of CV events and mortality
- Asymptomatic stage B HF: optimize treatment with interprofessional team to reduce progression to symptomatic (stage C) HF
- Asymptomatic stage B HF: start ACEi/ARBs and β-blockers to reduce risk for progression to symptomatic (stage C) HF
- Directed medical therapy for MI and symptomatic stage C HF: ACEi/ARBs, MRAs, angiotensin receptor/neprilysin inhibitor, β-blockers, and SGLT-2I, guideline-directed medical therapy for people without DM.

T1D and T2D
- Who is ketosis prone and/or those consuming ketogenic diets and using SGLT-2I should be educated on risks/signs of ketoacidosis and methods of risk management and provided with tools for accurate ketone measurement (ie, serum β-hydroxybutyrate)

Data from American Diabetes Association. 10. Cardiovascular disease and risk management: Standards of care in diabetes—2024. Diabetes Care. 2023;47(Supplement_1):S179-S218. https://doi.org/10.2337/dc24-S010; Joseph JJ, Deedwania P, Acharya T, et al. Comprehensive management of cardiovascular risk factors for adults with type 2 diabetes: A scientific statement from the American Heart Association. Circulation. 2022;145(9):e722-e759.

Table 3
Blood pressure management in the nonpregnant person with diabetes mellitus for cardiovascular risk factor reduction

Guidelines	Definition	Target BP	First-Line Agent	Dual Antihypertensive Therapy
American College of College/ American Heart Association (ACC/AHA)	130/80 mm Hg	<130/80 mm Hg	• Diuretics • ACEi or ARB • Calcium channel blockers (CCB)	>140/90 mm Hg
American Diabetes Association (ADA)	140/90 mm Hg	$\geq$130/80 mm Hg and <150/90 mm Hg	Start with 1 agent If NO Albuminuria or coronary artery disease (CAD): • ACEi or ARB • CCB • Diuretics	$\geq$150/90 mm Hg Start with 2 agents *If NO Albuminuria or CAD:* Start drug from 2 of 3 options • ACEi or ARB • CCB

(continued on next page)

Guidelines	Definition	Target BP	First-Line Agent	Dual Antihypertensive Therapy
			If Albuminuria or CAD • ACEi or ARB	• Diuretics *If Albuminuria or CAD* • ACEi or ARB and CCB or Diuretic

Table 3
(continued)

Abbreviations: ACEi, angiotensin-converting enzyme-inhibitor; ARB, angiotensin receptor blocker; BP, blood pressure; CV, cardiovascular.

*ACEi or ARB is suggested to treat hypertension for people with CAD or urine albumin-to-creatinine ratio 30 to 299 mg/g creatinine and strongly recommended for individuals with urine albumin-to-creatinine ratio $\geq$300 mg/g creatinine. Dihydropyridine CCB. Thiazide-like diuretic; long-acting agents shown to reduce CV events, such as chlorthalidone and indapamide, are preferred.[20]

Data from Refs[5,18,20]

Box 6

Initial lipid lowering management guidelines for reduction of cardiovascular risk factor reduction

Lifestyle and behavioral-focused approaches recommendation:
• Dietary Approaches to Stop Hypertension (DASH diet)
• Reduction of saturated fat and *trans* fat
• Increase of dietary n-3 fatty acids, viscous fiber, and plant stanol/sterol intake
• Increased physical activity to improve lipid profile
• Timely and aggressive lipid-lowering therapy is warranted for cardiovascular (CV) risk reduction
• Statins are the foundation
• 40 to 75 years old without ASCVD, use moderate-intensity statin therapy in addition to lifestyle therapy
• 20 to 39 years old with additional ASCVD risk factors, it may be reasonable to initiate statin therapy in addition to lifestyle therapy
• 40 to 75 years old at higher CV risk, including those with 1+ ASCVD risk, use high-intensity statin to reduce low-density lipoprotein (LDL) by $\geq$50% of baseline and target LDL goal of less than 70 mg/dL
• If established ASCVD, highest intensity statin tolerated; aim reducing LDL-C by at least 50% with more individualized approach for those greater than 75 years of age
• For primary prevention, moderate intensity statin should be considered
• Nonstatin therapies including ezetimibe, PCSK9 inhibitors, icosapent ethyl, bile acid resins, and fibrates should be considered after evaluation of risk, LDL-C after optimal statin therapy, and the presence of hypertriglyceridemia
• Fasting triglyceride levels $\geq$ 500 mg/dL: evaluate for secondary causes of hypertriglyceridemia and consider medical therapy to reduce the risk of pancreatitis
• Moderate hypertriglyceridemia (fasting or nonfasting triglycerides 175–499 mg/dL): address/treat lifestyle factors (obesity and metabolic syndrome), secondary factors (diabetes mellitus, chronic liver, or kidney disease and/or nephrotic syndrome, and hypothyroidism), and medications that raise triglycerides
• ASCVD or other CV risk factors on statin with controlled LDL but elevated triglycerides (135–499 mg/dL): add icosapent ethyl to reduce CV risk

Data from American Diabetes Association. 10. Cardiovascular disease and risk management: Standards of care in diabetes—2024. Diabetes Care. 2023;47(Supplement_1):S179-S218. https://doi.org/10.2337/dc24-S010; Joseph JJ, Deedwania P, Acharya T, et al. Comprehensive management of cardiovascular risk factors for adults with type 2 diabetes: A scientific statement from the American Heart Association. Circulation. 2022;145(9):e722-e759.

Box 7
Antithrombotic therapy management guidelines for cardiovascular risk reduction

- Aspirin 75 to 162 mg/day has a modest beneficial effect in primary prevention in nonelderly adults (50–70 years of age) with diabetes mellitus and increased cardiovascular (CV) risk based on additional clinical risk factors or imaging

- Documented aspirin allergy: use clopidogrel (75 mg/day)

- Length of treatment with dual antiplatelet therapy using low-dose aspirin and a P2Y12 inhibitor in after acute coronary syndrome or acute ischemic stroke/transient ischemic attack should be determined by an interprofessional team

- Combination therapy with aspirin plus low-dose rivaroxaban should be considered for stable coronary and/or peripheral artery disease and low bleeding risk to prevent major adverse limb and CV events

- Aspirin not recommended at low risk of ASCVD, as low benefit is likely to be outweighed by risk of bleeding

- Clinical judgment should be used for those at intermediate risk (younger individuals with one or more risk factors or older individuals with no risk factors) until further research is available

Data from American Diabetes Association. 10. Cardiovascular disease and risk management: Standards of care in diabetes—2024. Diabetes Care. 2023;47(Supplement_1):S179-S218. https://doi.org/10.2337/dc24-S010; Joseph JJ, Deedwania P, Acharya T, et al. Comprehensive management of cardiovascular risk factors for adults with type 2 diabetes: A scientific statement from the American Heart Association. Circulation. 2022;145(9):e722-e759.

Box 8
Diagnostic testing to assess subclinical cardiovascular disease

- In asymptomatic individuals: routine screening for coronary artery disease is not recommended, as it does not improve outcomes if ASCVD risk factors are treated

- Increased risk for development of asymptomatic cardiac structural/functional abnormalities (stage B HF) or symptomatic presentations (stage C HF): consider screening with (B-type natriuretic peptide (BNP) or N-terminal pro-BNP (NT-proBNP)) to facilitate prevention of stage C HF

- In asymptomatic age ≥ 50 years, microvascular disease in any location, foot complications or any end-organ damage from diabetes mellitus (DM): screening for peripheral artery disease (PAD) with ankle-brachial index testing is recommended. If DM duration ≥10 years: screening for PAD

- Coronary artery calcification

- Coronary artery computed tomography angiography

- Cardiac magnetic resonance imaging

- Stress testing

- Cardiac positron emission tomography

Summary:
- Many imaging tests can help with risk stratification but have limited date to support routine use
- Coronary artery calcium (CAC) scoring provides the most actionable triggers for lipid-lowering and antiplatelet therapy and is recommends escalation to high-intensity statin for CAC greater than 100

- CAC is reasonable in 30- to 39-year-old with long-standing DM and greater than 75-year-old adults if it would facilitate statin prescription

Aspirin also considered reasonable by National Lipid Association and Society of Cardiovascular Computed Tomography for CAC greater than 100.292

Ischemia testing in asymptomatic individuals with DM not currently recommended

Data from American Diabetes Association. 10. Cardiovascular disease and risk management: Standards of care in diabetes—2024. Diabetes Care. 2023;47(Supplement_1):S179-S218. https://doi.org/10.2337/dc24-S010; Joseph JJ, Deedwania P, Acharya T, et al. Comprehensive management of cardiovascular risk factors for adults with type 2 diabetes: A scientific statement from the American Heart Association. Circulation. 2022;145(9):e722-e759.

Table 4
Various treatment of coronary artery disease and angina

Medical Therapy to CAD and Angina
  *No antianginal medications have been shown to reduce morbidity or mortality in stable CAD Patients and have have similar results on reducing angina

Medical Therapy	Actions
Beta blockers (first line)	• Useful for vasodilating beta blocker effect with less side effects • Can elevate BG due to compensatory peripheral vasoconstriction which can lead to increased insulin resistance but also have some vasodilatory effects. Studies found a small but significant reduction in A1c weight loss and less progression to microalbuminuria
Calcium channel blockers (first line)	• Avoid nondihydropyridines • Helpful in persons with left ventricular dysfunction or with beta blockers
Long-acting nitrates	• Can build tolerance and endothelial dysfunction over time
Ranolazine	• No hemodynamic effects; moderate reduction in A1c • Reduces A1c by glucagon reduction • Both antianginal effect and glucose lowering effects are enhanced in poorly control PWD

Surgical Therapy to CAD and Angina
  * Both surgical and percutaneous revascularization outcomes are impaired in the setting of T2DM, with increased risk of both procedural complications and recurrent ischemic events.

Revascularization	• Coronary artery bypass graph (CABG) surgery is associated with lower MACEs compared with PCI • Use of the internal mammary artery to the anterior wall is an important driver of benefit of CABG • Typically achieve more complete revascularization with CABG vs PCI • Newest-generation drug-eluting stents have narrowed the gap between CABG and PCI

Abbreviations: BG, blood glucose; CAD, coronary artery disease; MACE, major adverse cardiovascular event; PCI, percutaneous coronary intervention; PWD, persons with diabetes; T2DM, type 2 diabetes mellitus.

Data from Arnold SV, Bhatt DL, Barsness GW, et al. Clinical management of stable coronary artery disease in patients with type 2 diabetes mellitus: a scientific statement from the American Heart Association. Circulation. 2020;141(19):e779-e806.

Box 6 will discuss initial lipid lowering management guidelines for reduction of CV risk factor reduction.[5,18]

Box 7 will discuss antithrombotic therapy management guidelines for CV risk reduction.[5,18]

Box 8 will discuss diagnostic testing to assess subclinical CVD.[5,18]

Management of Stable Angina

Approximately about one-third of people with stable CAD will report chronic angina despite the new medical and surgical treatments. Despite advances in interventions that prevent and slow the progression of atherosclerosis and revascularization technologies to reduce myocardial ischemia, about one-third of patients with stable CAD reports chronic angina.[21] PWD many times have diffuse coronary disease and their angina often is under treated and even missed.[22]

Table 4 discusses the various treatments of CAD and angina.[23]

SUMMARY

In summary, many diabetes and CV organizations develop very robust treatment standards, often on a yearly basis to give guidance for CV risk reduction for PWD. CV complication reductions have been well researched, and current recommendations of lifestyle modifications, lipid lowering measures, blood pressure reduction, and person-centered care goals with targeted glycemic goals will see benefits by following these evidence-based guidelines. However, most of these guidelines for goal-directed therapy were tested on persons with T2D. Age and length of time with diabetes is very a significant factor, followed by A1c, blood pressure measurements, and low-density lipoprotein cholesterol (LDL-C) especially after 15 to 20 years from initial diagnosis severely impacts CV risk. Research has found that simply the variable of hyperglycemia may affect CV risk in persons with T1D more so than in those with T2D.[24–27] Therefore, medical providers often need to extrapolate the T2D data to develop a mutual patient care decisions to collaboratively care for persons with T1D.

CLINICS CARE POINTS

- Diabetes regardless of the type, affects over 38 million persons in the United States.

- Regardless of all the new technologies and pharmacologic interventions, PWD still has a very high percentage of CV disease.

- Professional medical organizations including the American Diabetes Association and the American Heart Association publish robust research discoveries in yearly guidelines and scientific papers to offer more pathways to reduce complications of CV disease in PWD.

- These recent guidelines include updated efficacy and use for many new CV disease reduction diabetes medications such as DPP-4 inhibitors, glucagon-like peptide-1 receptor agonist, SGLT-2 inhibitors, strategies to reduce blood pressure, lipids levels, thrombus formation, CV diagnostic testing, facilitating positive health behaviors, and understanding up-to-date management for PWD and stable angina.

DISCLOSURE

The author was a certified Medtronic insulin pump and sensor trainer in the past but has not trained patients in more than 5 years.

REFERENCES

1. Centers for Disease Control and Prevention. National Diabetes Statistics Report. 2024, Available at: https://www.cdc.gov/diabetes/php/data-research/?CDC_AAref_Val=https://www.cdc.gov/diabetes/data/statistics-report/index.html.
2. American Diabetes Association. 2. Diagnosis and classification of diabetes: standards of care in diabetes—2024. Diabetes Care 2024;47(Supplement_1): S20–42.
3. Yu MG, Gordin D, Fu J, et al. Protective factors and the pathogenesis of complications in diabetes. Endocr Rev 2023;45(2):227–52.
4. Yun J-S, Ko S-H. Current trends in epidemiology of cardiovascular disease and cardiovascular risk management in type 2 diabetes. Metabolism 2021;123: 154838.
5. American Diabetes Association. 10. Cardiovascular disease and risk management: standards of care in diabetes—2024. Diabetes Care 2023;47(Supplement_1): S179–218.
6. Narayan KMV. Glycemic control and cardiovascular disease in patients with type 1 diabetes. Clin Diabetes 2006;24(2):88–9.
7. Cheng YJ, Imperatore G, Geiss LS, et al. Trends and disparities in cardiovascular mortality among US adults with and without self-reported diabetes, 1988–2015. Diabetes Care 2018;41(11):2306–15.
8. Einarson TR, Acs A, Ludwig C, et al. Prevalence of cardiovascular disease in type 2 diabetes: a systematic literature review of scientific evidence from across the world in 2007–2017. Cardiovasc Diabetol 2018;17:1–19.
9. National Institutes of Health. DCCT and EDIC: the diabetes control and complication trial and followup study. 2008.
10. Epidemiology of diabetes interventions complications research group. Epidemiology of diabetes interventions and complications (EDIC): design, implementation, and preliminary results of a long-term follow-up of the diabetes control and complications trial cohort. Diabetes Care 1999;22(1):99.
11. Schofield J, Ho J, Soran H. Cardiovascular risk in type 1 diabetes mellitus. Diabetes Ther 2019;10(3):773–89.
12. Huang Y, Cai X, Mai W, et al. Association between prediabetes and risk of cardiovascular disease and all cause mortality: systematic review and meta-analysis. Bmj 2016;355.
13. Ali MK, Bullard KM, Saydah S, et al. Cardiovascular and renal burdens of prediabetes in the USA: analysis of data from serial cross-sectional surveys, 1988–2014. Lancet Diabetes Endocrinol 2018;6(5):392–403.
14. Brannick B, Wynn A, Dagogo-Jack S. Prediabetes as a toxic environment for the initiation of microvascular and macrovascular complications. Exp Biol Med 2016; 241(12):1323–31.
15. Zand A, Ibrahim K, Patham B. Prediabetes: why should we care? Methodist DeBakey Cardiovascular Journal 2018;14(4):289.
16. Lawal Y, Bello F, Kaoje YS. Prediabetes deserves more attention: a review. Clin Diabetes 2020;38(4):328–38.
17. Cai X, Zhang Y, Li M, et al. Association between prediabetes and risk of all cause mortality and cardiovascular disease: updated meta-analysis. BMJ 2020;370.
18. Joseph JJ, Deedwania P, Acharya T, et al. Comprehensive management of cardiovascular risk factors for adults with type 2 diabetes: a scientific statement from the American Heart Association. Circulation 2022;145(9):e722–59.

19. American Diabetes Association. 5. facilitating positive health behaviors and well-being to improve health outcomes: standards of care in diabetes—2024. Diabetes Care 2023;47(Supplement_1):S77–110.
20. De Boer IH, Bangalore S, Benetos A, et al. Diabetes and hypertension: a position statement by the American Diabetes Association. Diabetes Care 2017;40(9):1273–84.
21. Kureshi F, Shafiq A, Arnold SV, et al. The prevalence and management of angina among patients with chronic coronary artery disease across US outpatient cardiology practices: insights from the Angina Prevalence and Provider Evaluation of Angina Relief (APPEAR) study. Clin Cardiol 2017;40(1):6–10.
22. Qintar M, Spertus JA, Gosch KL, et al. Effect of angina under-recognition on treatment in outpatients with stable ischaemic heart disease. European Heart Journal–Quality of Care and Clinical Outcomes 2016;2(3):208–14.
23. Arnold SV, Bhatt DL, Barsness GW, et al. Clinical management of stable coronary artery disease in patients with type 2 diabetes mellitus: a scientific statement from the American Heart Association. Circulation 2020;141(19):e779–806.
24. Writing team for the diabetes control and complications trial/epidemiology for diabetes interventions and complications research group. Sustained effect of intensive treatment of type 1 diabetes mellitus on development and progression of diabetic nephropathy: the epidemiology of diabetes interventions and complications (EDIC) study. JAMA, J Am Med Assoc 2003;290(16):2159.
25. Colom C, Rull A, Sanchez-Quesada JL, et al. Cardiovascular disease in type 1 diabetes mellitus: epidemiology and management of cardiovascular risk. J Clin Med 2021;10(8). https://doi.org/10.3390/jcm10081798.
26. Lind M, Svensson A-M, Kosiborod M, et al. Glycemic control and excess mortality in type 1 diabetes. N Engl J Med 2014;371(21):1972–82.
27. Bebu I, Braffett BH, Pop-Busui R, et al. The relationship of blood glucose with cardiovascular disease is mediated over time by traditional risk factors in type 1 diabetes: the DCCT/EDIC study. Diabetologia 2017;60(10):2084–91.

Diabetes Management in the Critical Care Setting
Insulin Infusions

Marjorie R. Ortiz, MSN, RN, AGPCNP-BC, BC-ADM

KEYWORDS

- Intravenous insulin infusion • Inpatient hyperglycemia management
- Critical care nursing • Insulin drip

KEY POINTS

- Hyperglycemia in critical care patients is common and requires early intervention.
- Insulin infusions are used to reach glucose targets without increasing the risk of hypoglycemia in critically ill patients.
- Nurses play a key role in initiating, managing, and transitioning off insulin infusions in critically ill patients.

BACKGROUND

Diabetes mellitus affects a large portion of the population in the United States. The Centers for Disease Control estimated that in 2022, 38.4 million adults, or 11.6% of the US population, had diabetes, with another 22.8% of adults undiagnosed. Additionally, it is estimated that 38% of the adult US population has prediabetes.[1] Patients with diabetes commonly have comorbid conditions such as high blood pressure and high cholesterol, and may develop complications such as kidney disease, microvascular complications, coronary artery disease, and cerebrovascular disease if diabetes is left untreated or uncontrolled. People with diabetes have higher rates of hospitalization compared with the general population due to these comorbid conditions and complications.[2]

Diabetes is common in hospitalized patients, with recent data showing that nearly a quarter of hospitalized patients have a diagnosis of diabetes.[2] Hyperglycemia can occur in patients with an existing diagnosis of diabetes, those with undiagnosed diabetes, or those with no diagnosis of diabetes, who may experience hyperglycemia secondary to physiologic stress, medications, and other external factors. If hyperglycemia persists, patients are at higher risk of adverse outcomes, longer length of

Department of Endocrine Neoplasia and Hormonal Disorders, The University of Texas MD Anderson Cancer Center, Houston, Texas, USA
E-mail address: MOrtiz2@mdanderson.org

hospital stay, and mortality.[3] For these reasons, it is important to identify patients at risk for uncontrolled glucose levels while hospitalized and to intervene early for the best possible outcomes. Nurses play a key role in identifying and treating patients with hyperglycemia in the hospital.

DEFINITIONS AND GLUCOSE TARGETS

On admission to the hospital, patients should be evaluated for hyperglycemia risk factors. A hemoglobin A1C level of greater than 6.4% is diagnostic of diabetes and indicates that hyperglycemia preceded the hospitalization[4]; thus, glucose monitoring should be initiated on admission. Hyperglycemia can also occur in patients without a history of hyperglycemia. Other causes of hyperglycemia include—but are not limited to—stress, medication (eg, steroids), enteral and parenteral nutrition, and omission of home diabetes medications.[5] Challenges to glucose management in critically ill patients include their unstable hemodynamics, various medications, and nutritional needs.[6] A list of common factors affecting glucose levels in hospitalized patients can be found in **Box 1**.

Hyperglycemia in the hospitalized patient is defined as a glucose level greater than 140 mg/dL.[6] Glucose-lowering therapy should be initiated in hospitalized patients when glucose is persistently over 180 mg/dL. Lower glucose targets of 110 to 140 mg/dL have been shown to benefit postsurgical patients if the target can be achieved without causing hypoglycemia[6]; however, tight glucose control in critically ill patients has been shown to increase risk of hypoglycemia, which in turn increases morbidity and mortality.[7] In most critical care patients, a glucose target of 140 to 180 mg/dL is appropriate; a glucose target of less than 110 mg/dL is generally not recommended[7,8] (**Box 2**).

INSULIN INFUSIONS: USES, INDICATIONS, MONITORING

Glucose control in the critical care setting can be achieved through several methods, depending on the clinical situation of the patient. When the resources are available, it is beneficial to involve the expertise of a specialized diabetes management team to assist in the care of this patient population.[6] Insulin is the preferred medication used to treat hyperglycemia due to its ability to rapidly lower glucose levels and the ease of dose adjustments. However, as a high-risk medication, insulin necessitates precise monitoring and standardized protocols to mitigate potential risks such as hypoglycemia. The use of sliding-scale/correction-scale subcutaneous insulin injections alone to treat hyperglycemia is outdated and not beneficial in managing glucose levels.[9] If

---

Box 1
Factors affecting glycemic control in hospitalized patients

- Glucose control prior to admission
- Change in nutritional status (oral diet, enteral nutrition, parenteral nutrition)
- Vasopressors
- Corticosteroids
- Sliding-scale insulin used as monotherapy
- Omission of home diabetes medications
- Hepatic or renal impairment

Box 2
Critical care glucose targets

- Hyperglycemia = glucose greater than 140 mg/dL
- ICU glucose targets for most patients: 140 to 180 mg/dL
- ICU glucose targets for postsurgical patients: 110 to 140 mg/dL (if benefit outweighs hypoglycemia risk)
- ICU glucose targets of less than 110 mg/dL are not recommended

---

subcutaneous insulin is used, it is preferred to use a basal bolus insulin regimen instead of sliding-scale insulin alone. The use of a continuous intravenous (IV) insulin infusion is the most effective way to manage glucose levels in the critical care setting. Studies have shown that continuous insulin infusion protocols are associated with better glucose control while also avoiding hypoglycemia.[9]

Regular insulin (Humulin R or Novolin R) is the type of insulin that is used in IV insulin infusions. It can be administered through a central line or a peripheral IV. Insulin infusions consist of 100 units of regular insulin mixed in 100 mL of normal saline. Insulin infusion protocols differ on the starting dose of the insulin infusion and on whether a bolus of insulin should be given at the initiation of the continuous infusion.

Continuous insulin infusions may be used in a variety of situations, from hyperglycemia management to simply reduce glucose levels to hyperglycemia emergencies such as diabetic ketoacidosis and hyperglycemic hyperosmolar state. Other situations in which continuous insulin infusions are appropriate are listed in **Box 3**. In hyperglycemic emergencies, the continuous insulin infusion protocol is used to reduce glucose levels as well as to correct acid-base balance and electrolyte abnormalities.[10] The short half-life of IV insulin allows for rapid dose adjustments.

Insulin infusion protocols vary from institution to institution and should be based on validated written or computerized protocols, with specific instructions regarding adjustments in the infusion rates based on glycemic changes and rates of change.[12] Insulin infusion protocols also vary depending on the indication for insulin infusion as well as whether an initial bolus of IV insulin is given at the initiation of the infusion. While

---

Box 3
Common indications for continuous insulin infusions[10,11]

- Diabetic ketoacidosis/hyperglycemic hyperosmolar state
- Critical care illness
- Postcardiac surgery
- Prolonged NPO status in insulin-deficient patients
- Perioperative glucose management in critically ill patients
- Post-organ transplantation
- Stroke
- Poor glucose control on subcutaneous insulin
- Deducing insulin requirements before converting to subcutaneous insulin
- Labor and delivery

---

no specific protocol will be discussed here, the underlying components of insulin infusion protocols are universal to ensure a safe and effective delivery method. Insulin infusion protocols should include the following.[11]

- Clear glucose targets appropriate for the situation
- Clear indications when insulin infusion should be implemented
- Management of insulin infusions by nursing staff and straightforward implementation
- Clear, specific instructions for glucose monitoring and titration
- Titration based on both the glucose level and rate of change
- Low risk of hypoglycemia and a hypoglycemia protocol should this occur
- Achievement of blood glucose target and maintenance of glucose level within the target range
- A plan for transition to subcutaneous insulin

Nurses play a key role in the management of patients on insulin infusions. A list of common responsibilities for nursing staff in critical care patients on insulin infusions can be found in **Box 4**.

CURRENT GUIDELINES

The Society of Critical Care Medicine, American Diabetes Association, and American Association of Clinical Endocrinology all recommend initiation of insulin infusions in critically ill patients at glucose thresholds over 180 mg/dL.[6,8,13,14] Contributing factors to hyperglycemia must be considered and altered if needed, such as fluids, nutrition, or medications.

The Society of Critical Care Medicine updated its guidelines for IV insulin management in critically ill patients in 2024; these are summarized here and found in **Table 1**. It is suggested that continuous IV insulin infusion, rather than subcutaneous insulin, be used in the acute management of hyperglycemia in critically ill patients. While IV insulin infusions do require higher nursing workload, more monitoring, and frequent interruptions to the patient, better glycemic control can be achieved with insulin infusions rather than subcutaneous insulin. Additionally, variability in absorption of subcutaneous

---

Box 4
Nursing responsibilities for patients on insulin infusions

- Assess patient for underlying diabetes: type 1 versus type 2 versus drug-induced
- Assist in identifying patients in need of IV insulin infusion
- Understand indication for insulin infusion
- Review insulin infusion protocol and orders
- Review labs prior to initiation of insulin infusion and replace electrolytes if needed according to orders
- Document blood glucose levels and insulin dose adjustments in a standardized location in the medical record according to the individual institution's procedure
- Be aware of signs/symptoms and treatment of hypoglycemia
- Educate patient/family on indication for insulin infusion, frequency of glucose checks and labs
- Ensure orders are carried out for transition to subcutaneous insulin; ensure patient receives basal insulin prior to discontinuation of the infusion.

Table 1
Society of Critical Care Medicine guidelines for insulin infusions 2024

Critically Ill Adults	Critically Ill Children
• Providers should initiate treatment of hyperglycemia in critically ill patients with glucose persistently over 180 mg/dL. • Glycemic management protocols with low hypoglycemia risk should be used. • Hypoglycemia requires immediate treatment. • Lower glucose targets of 80–139 mg/dL are not recommended as compared with targets of 140–200 mg/dL due to risk of hypoglycemia in critically ill patients. • Continuous IV insulin infusion is recommended over subcutaneous insulin in the acute management of critically ill adults. • Frequent glucose monitoring (every hour) is recommended during times of glycemic variability.	• Providers should initiate treatment of hyperglycemia in critically ill children with glucose persistently over 180 mg/dL. • Glycemic management protocols with low hypoglycemia risk should be used. • Hypoglycemia requires immediate treatment. • Lower glucose targets of 80–139 mg/dL are not recommended as compared with targets of 140–200 mg/dL due to risk of hypoglycemia in critically ill patients. • No recommendation is made for the use of continuous IV insulin over subcutaneous insulin, but most experts on the panel use continuous insulin infusions as therapy of choice. • No recommendation for frequency of blood glucose monitoring, but most experts note that frequent glucose monitoring ($\leq$1-h intervals) are used in children being treated with continuous IV insulin. • Explicit decision support tools are suggested for use in pediatric patients being treated with continuous IV insulin infusions.

Abbreviation: IV, intravenous.

insulin with the use of vasopressors, poor perfusion, or edema makes IV insulin more appropriate for critically ill patients.[8]

Insulin infusion protocols should have a low hypoglycemic risk profile. Should hypoglycemia occur, it should be treated promptly. It is not advised to titrate an insulin infusion to a more intense, lower glucose target of 80 to 139 mg/dL, as this increases the risk of hypoglycemia.

Glucose monitoring while on continuous insulin infusions should be frequent—at least every hour during times of glycemic variability. Frequent glucose monitoring via point-of-care testing improves glycemic control, reduces hypoglycemia and enables early recognition of rapidly changing glucose levels. With frequent glucose monitoring comes increased workload for nursing staff and increased discomfort to the patients. . In patients who are clinically stable with a lower risk of hypoglycemia, the frequency of glucose monitoring may be decreased. As an alternative to point of care glucose testing, continuous glucose monitors are used in certain institutions to reduce the frequency of point-of-care glucose testing Point-of-care testing is still required for calibration of these devices. The use of continuous glucose monitors decreases nurse workload and is as effective as point-of-care glucose testing.[15] Continuous glucose monitor use in hospitalized patients requires specialized training, approval by the institution, and established policies and procedures, which can vary between institutions. The final recommendation for adult patients in the critical care setting is that a protocol with explicit decision support tools be used in adults who are being treated with IV insulin infusion.[8]

RISKS OF INSULIN INFUSIONS: HYPOGLYCEMIA

Frequent glucose monitoring during insulin infusion allows for early recognition of hypoglycemia. Insulin infusion protocols should include a hypoglycemia protocol within the orders to allow for nursing staff to treat hypoglycemia immediately with standing orders. A hypoglycemia protocol within the insulin infusion protocol should include specific instructions for discontinuing or decreasing the rate of the IV insulin infusion and starting continuous dextrose IV fluids or IV push. If the protocol dictates to stop the insulin infusion, there should be clear instructions on when the infusion should be resumed and at what rate. Nursing staff should be aware of the signs and symptoms of hypoglycemia, which most commonly include diaphoresis, tremors, nausea, confusion, and in severe hypoglycemia, loss of consciousness.

RISKS OF INSULIN INFUSIONS: HYPOKALEMIA

Insulin drives glucose into the cell. As this occurs, potassium follows the glucose, thereby decreasing serum potassium levels. Hypokalemia is associated with increased mortality. It is important to replete potassium prior to administering IV insulin to avoid arrhythmias and respiratory muscle weakness.[10] Nursing staff should monitor labs before initiation of the insulin infusion. Laboratory studies are frequently monitored while patients are receiving IV insulin infusions to monitor for electrolyte abnormalities such as these.

RISKS OF INSULIN INFUSIONS: CEREBRAL EDEMA

Cerebral edema is a very rare yet devastating complication of the rapid correction of hyperglycemia and electrolyte abnormalities during hyperglycemic crisis, and carries a mortality rate of 20% to 40%.[10] It most commonly occurs in children and is very rare in adults. The rapid shift in intracellular and extracellular fluid levels that can accompany rapid correction of hyperglycemia contributes to the development of this life-threatening complication.[10] Nurses and care team providers should be aware of this potential complication and monitor patients for neurologic changes. Frequent glucose monitoring and laboratory monitoring are necessary to ensure gradual correction of severe hyperglycemia and acidosis in patients presenting in hyperglycemic crises.[11]

TRANSITIONING TO SUBCUTANEOUS INSULIN INJECTIONS

Proper transition from insulin infusion to subcutaneous insulin is important to ensure continued adequate glucose control and prevent rebound hyperglycemia. Transitioning from IV insulin infusions to subcutaneous insulin injections requires careful planning and preparation. Critical care providers and/or members of the diabetes management team will determine the appropriate time to transition to subcutaneous insulin. Indications for insulin infusion transition include stable glucose measurements for 4 to 6 hours on the infusion, normal anion gap, normalization in electrolytes, hemodynamic stability (ie, not receiving vasopressors), stable nutrition, and stable insulin infusion rates[11,16] (**Table 2**).

It is recommended that a transition protocol be used to assist the transition from IV insulin infusion to subcutaneous insulin injections.[16] Dosing for subcutaneous insulin can be calculated in several ways: (1) based on the IV insulin infusion rate during the prior 6 to 8 hours during which glucose levels were stable and not changing rapidly; (2) based on prior home insulin dose; or (3) weight-based dosing.

Basal insulin has an onset of action of several hours and thus requires some overlap with insulin infusion, at a minimum 1 to 2 hours. Basal insulin should be injected at least 2 hours prior to the discontinuation of the insulin infusion. Some studies show that basal insulin can be given concomitantly with the insulin infusion. This in turn would help decrease the length of time on the insulin infusion, decrease the risk of

Table 2
Indications and contraindications for transition to subcutaneous insulin

Indications	Contraindications
• Stable glucose for at least 4–6 h	• High variability in infusion rates
• Normal anion gap and electrolytes	• Highly variable glucose levels
• Hemodynamic stability	• High insulin infusion rates on the infusion
• Not on vasopressors	• No resolution of diabetic ketoacidosis
• Stable nutrition	
• Stable intravenous drip rates	

rebound hyperglycemia, and decrease the length of stay.[16] It is specifically important for patients with type 1 diabetes or insulin deficiency to receive basal (long-acting) insulin before the discontinuation of the insulin infusion. Premature discontinuation of the IV insulin infusion prior to injecting basal insulin can result in not only rebound hyperglycemia but also diabetic ketoacidosis in patients with insulin deficiency or type 1 diabetes.

NURSING CONSIDERATIONS AND TAKE-HOME POINTS

Hospitalized patients, especially those with a preexisting diagnosis of diabetes mellitus, should be assessed on admission for hyperglycemia, with glucose monitoring and early intervention if indicated. Critically ill patients in the intensive care setting present unique challenges for glucose control due to factors such as unstable hemodynamics, medication side effects, and nutritional needs. Continuous IV insulin infusion is the preferred method for managing hyperglycemia in the critical care setting due to its rapid action and ease of adjustment. Nurses play a vital role in glucose management, from assessment and insulin infusion protocol adherence to patient education and monitoring for complications. By following evidence-based guidelines and with collaboration within interdisciplinary teams, nurses can optimize patient outcomes and minimize the risks associated with hyperglycemia in critical care patients.

DISCLOSURE

The author has nothing to disclose.

REFERENCES

1. Centers for Disease Control and Prevention. National diabetes statistics report. Available at: https://www.cdc.gov/diabetes/data/statistics-report/index.html. Accessed November 29, 2023.
2. Zhang Y, Bullard KM, Imperatore G, et al. Proportions and trends of adult hospitalizations with diabetes, United States, 2000–2018. Diabetes Res Clin Pract 2022;187:109862.
3. Pasquel JF, Lansang MC, Dhatariya K, et al. Management of diabetes and hyperglycaemia in the hospital. Lancet Diabetes Endocrinol 2021;9(3):174–88.
4. American Diabetes Association Professional Practice Committee. 2. Diagnosis and classification of diabetes: standards of care in diabetes—2024. Diabetes Care 2024;47(Supplement1):S20–42.
5. Clement S, Braithwaite SS, Magee MF, et al. Management of diabetes and hyperglycemia in hospitals. Diabetes Care 2004;27:553–91.

6. American Diabetes Association Professional Practice Committee. 16. Diabetes care in the hospital: standards of care in diabetes—2024. Diabetes Care 2024; 47(Supplement1):S295–306.

7. Griesdale DE, de Souza RJ, van Dam RM, et al. Intensive insulin therapy and mortality among critically ill patients: a meta-analysis including NICE-SUGAR study data. CMAJ (Can Med Assoc J) 2009;180(8):821–7.

8. Honarmand K, Sirimaturos M, Hirshberg E, et al. Society of critical care medicine guidelines on glycemic control for critically ill children and adults 2024. Crit Care Med 2024;52(4):e161–81.

9. Tran KK, Kibert JL, Telford ED, et al. Intravenous insulin infusion protocol compared with subcutaneous insulin for the management of hyperglycemia in critically ill adults. Ann Pharmacother 2019;53(9):894–8.

10. Kitabchi AE, Umpierrez GE, Miles JM, et al. Hyperglycemic crises in adult patients with diabetes. Diabetes Care 2009;32(7):1335–43.

11. Kelly JL. Continuous insulin infusion: when, where, and how? Diabetes Spectr 2014;27(3):218.

12. Hohn S. Implementing a computerized inpatient insulin protocol system. AADE in Practice. 2013;1(6):26–8.

13. Blonde L, Umpierrez GE, Reddy SS, et al. American Association of Clinical Endocrinology Clinical Practice Guideline: developing a diabetes mellitus comprehensive care plan-2022 update. Endocr Pract 2022;28:923–1049.

14. Moghissi ES, Korytkowski MT, DiNardo M, et al. American Association of Clinical Endocrinologists and American Diabetes Association consensus statement on inpatient glycemic control. Diabetes Care 2009;32(6):1119–31.

15. Boom DT, Sechterberger MK, Rijkenberg S, et al. Insulin treatment guided by subcutaneous continuous glucose monitoring compared to frequent point-of-care measurement in critically ill patients: a randomized controlled trial. Crit Care 2014;18:453.

16. Umpierrez GE, Hellman R, Korytkowski MT, et al. Management of hyperglycemia in hospitalized patients in non-critical care setting: an Endocrine Society clinical practice guideline. J Clin Endocrinol Metab 2012;97:16–38.

Current Medical Nutrition Therapy Recommendations for the Person with Diabetes

Celia Ann Levesque, APRN, NP-C, CNS-BC, CDCES, BC-ADM

KEYWORDS

- Diabetes • Nutrition • Malnutrition • Medical nutrition therapy • Dietary methods
- Clear liquid diet • Enteral nutrition • Parenteral nutrition

KEY POINTS

- Individualized medical nutrition therapy for the person with diabetes should be individualized to meet nutrition requirements, glycemic goals, and desired body weight.
- The nutrition method should consider patient preferences on eating patterns and types of foods as much as possible.
- Hospitalized patients with diabetes are at risk for malnutrition and should be screened for malnourishment.
- Hospitalized patients with diabetes will need to have close glucose monitoring and a custom diabetes medication plan depending on the meal plan such as regular diet, controlled carbohydrate diet, carbohydrate counting, clear liquid diet, enteral nutrition, and/or parental nutrition.
- Nutrition assessments, creation of an individualized dietary method, and patient education should be carried out by a registered dietitian knowledgeable in assessing nutrition status and creating a healthy meal plan that the patients follow.

INTRODUCTION

The American Diabetes Association (ADA) does not have specific macronutrient or micronutrient recommendations for the person with diabetes (PWD); therefore, the term 'American Diabetes Association' diet should no longer be used. The word "diet" is often associated with omission of entire food groups, strict calorie restriction, feeling deprived, being hungry, and not being sustainable long-term. The ADA recommends individualized medical nutrition therapy (MNT) for the PWD be based on nutritional needs. The emphasis has shifted from exact macronutrients and micronutrients to dietary patterns with a focus on nutrient-dense foods with amounts to achieve and maintain weight, glycemic, lipid, and blood pressure goals.[1]

Department of Endocrine Neoplasia and Hormonal Disorders, The University of Texas MD Anderson Cancer Center, Houston, TX, USA
E-mail address: clevesqu@mdanderson.org

Crit Care Nurs Clin N Am 37 (2025) 75–83
https://doi.org/10.1016/j.cnc.2024.09.002
0899-5885/25/© 2024 Elsevier Inc. All rights reserved, including those for text and data mining, AI training, and similar technologies.

ccnursing.theclinics.com

Nutrient dense foods include:

- Non starchy vegetables
- Whole fruits
- Legumes
- Whole grains
- Nuts/seeds
- Low fat dairy products

Foods that the amounts should be limited:

- Meat
- Sugar-sweetened beverages
- Sweets
- Refined grains
- Ultra-processed foods[1]

The overall goal is to prevent, delay, or slow progression of long-term diabetes related complications. The patient should be able to eat the foods they love with moderation of the foods that cause problems with blood glucose, lipids, blood pressure, and/or weight. MNT design and education should be provided by a registered dietitian with knowledge and experience in diabetes. The meal plan should be developed with the PWD and be adjusted as needed based on patient preferences and change in patient circumstances.[2,3] If the PWD is overweight or has obesity, the recommendation is to lose a minimum of 5% body weight. Total carbohydrate grams per meal may need to be adjusted based on postprandial glucose values. High fiber sources of carbohydrate should be included with the goal of at least 14 g of fiber per 1000 calories. Protein consumption in people with type 2 diabetes (T2D) may increase insulin response so if the person with T2D has hypoglycemia, then it should be treated with a simple carbohydrate that is low in fat and protein. Skytte and colleagues studied a carbohydrate-reduced, high protein diet in patients with T2D and found the diet improved hemoglobin A1c (HbA1c) and liver fat in patients whose weight was stable.[4] In people with type 1 diabetes (T1D), protein and fat may contribute to postprandial hyperglycemia so some with T1D need to factor protein and fat with carbohydrate grams when deciding on the prandial dose of insulin. The fat intake source should come from monounsaturated, polyunsaturated, and/or long-chain fatty acids. Alcohol should be limited to 1 drink equivalent per day or less in women and 2 drink equivalents per day or less in men. Sodium should be limited to less than 2300 mg per day. The use of non-nutritive sweeteners may be used in moderation. There is no evidence to support the use of supplements for PWD without nutritional deficiencies.[1]

DIETARY METHODS FOR MEAL PLANNING

There are different methods for meal planning but are not well-studied and studies had varied results on the impact of certain diets on HbA1c levels. A variety of eating patterns are acceptable to manage diabetes. The healthcare provider should emphasize non-starchy vegetables, minimize added sugars and refined grains, and choose whole foods over processed foods.

Common meal plan approaches include:

- Fixed carbohydrate meals/snacks
- Simplified carbohydrate counting tool
- Meal size estimation (small, medium, and large)

- Plate method
- Intermittent fasting or time-restricted
- Continuous calorie restricted
- Low or very-low carbohydrate diets
- Low or very-low fat diets
- Mediterranean-style
- Dietary Approaches to Stop Hypertension
- Paleo
- Vegetarian or vegan
- United States Department of Agriculture Dietary guidelines for Americans
- Use of partial meal replacements
- Insulin to carbohydrate ratio
- Total available glucose method of carbohydrate counting

PATIENTS WITH DIABETES USING PRANDIAL INSULIN

PWD who use prandial insulin should receive education about matching the prandial insulin dose to the amount of carbohydrate that will be consumed. Builes-Montano and colleagues looked at the efficacy and safety of carbohydrate counting versus other forms of dietary advice for patients with T1D and found carbohydrate counting significantly reduces HbA1c.[5] Some PWD will also need to consider the effects of protein and fat on blood glucose. Fat intake contributes to postprandial insulin resistance. High protein intake in people with T1D may contribute to postprandial hyperglycemia. If PWD are on a fixed dose of insulin at meal, the focus should be on a fixed amount of carbohydrate at the meals.

NUTRITION THERAPY IN HOSPITALIZED PATIENTS WITH DIABETES

Nutritional needs in the hospital are often different compared to home. The hospitalized PWD should have an assessment for nutritional status and a plan to meet the nutritional requirements.[3,6]

Malnutrition, especially in older patients, increases the risk for adverse medical outcomes and is commonly unrecognized. The prevalence of malnutrition in intensive care unit (ICU) patients is 40%. Patients over age 65 y have a 1.2 to 2.3 times higher risk for malnutrition than those younger.[3,6] Risk factors for the development of malnourishment include inadequate nutrient intake due to a variety of causes such as decreased oral intake, increased caloric requirements due to illness/disease, and decreased absorption of nutrients. Patients with overweight or obesity can have malnourishment.

Patients with malnutrition are at increased risk for:

- Impaired immune function
- Delayed healing
- Infection
- Decreased body mass leading to weakened respiratory muscles and decreased ventilatory drive
- Increased length-of-stay
- Hypoglycemia
- Mortality
- Functional decline
- Rehospitalization
- Discharge to skilled nursing facility or rehabilitation[3,6,7]

Common nutrition issues in hospitalized PWD:

- Poor appetite, altered taste, nausea, and/or vomiting
- Acute medical illness increasing the metabolic demands due to catabolic stress
- Hyperglycemia leading to glycosuria and calorie loss
- Limited food choice/patient does not like the food choices on the menu
- Lack of culturally specific food
- Dietary restrictions in the hospital such as low sodium that the patient does not like the food choices
- Some hospitals have inflexible meal times[3,6]

NUTRITIONAL SCREENING TOOLS

Many nutrition screening tools exist.[8] Ideally, the tool is easy to apply, cost-effective, identifies who needs an assessment, and is accepted by the patient and clinical staff. There is no standard nutritional screening tool agreed upon. Most tools include body mass index (BMI), history of weight loss, food intake, and potential nutritional decline due to current illness. The American Society for Parenteral and Enteral nutrition and the Academy of Nutrition and Dietetics recommend that malnutrition should be diagnosed if the patient has 2 of the following.

- Weight loss
- Low energy intake
- Loss of subcutaneous fat
- Fluid accumulation
- Muscle mass loss
- Weakened grip strength[6]

The Global Leadership Initiative on malnutrition recommends the diagnosis of malnutrition be based on 1 or more of the following:

- Unintentional weight loss
- Low BMI and/or loss of muscle mass
- Decreased food intake
- Inflammation or disease burden

Common screening tools include.

- The Mini Nutritional Assessment Short Form
- The Malnutrition Universal Screening Tool
- Simplified Nutritional Appetite Questionnaire
- Geriatric Nutritional Risk Index
- Malnutrition Universal Screen Tool
- Malnutrition Screening Tool
- Determine your Health Nutritional Screening Initiative checklist
- Nutritional Status Score
- Rapid Screen
- Subjective Global Assessment[3,8]

Nutrition goals for hospitalized patients with diabetes mellitus include:

- Meet glycemic goals
- Avoidance of hypoglycemia
- Avoidance of significant and prolonged hyperglycemia
- Meet calorie and nutrient requirements[9]

MNT for PWD is creating an individualized meal plan based on a nutrition assessment by a trained registered dietitian to meet nutrition requirements taking into consideration food preferences of the PWD. The goal of MNT is to meet caloric demands, meet glycemic goals for hospitalization, accommodate food preferences if possible, and provide a discharge plan.[9]

Nutrition Assessment

If a patient cannot consume 60% or more of nutrition requirements for 5 d in patients in ICU or in 7 to 14 d in the general population, then they are a candidate for nutrition support (3). Most hospitalized PWD require 25 to 35 calories per kg per d (1800 – 2000 calories per d). Most need approximately 200 g of carbohydrate per day.

BODY MASS INDEX

BMI is commonly used in the screening tools to assess nutrition status, but it may not be accurate in every person. It may underestimate in older people with malnutrition and overestimate in younger people well-nourished. It also is not an indicator of protein-energy malnutrition. The screening tools using BMI to diagnose malnutrition do not have a standard number to diagnose malnutrition. Using BMI may miss some patients with malnutrition in patients who are older with higher BMI. Measuring limb circumference is commonly used to assess lean body and fat mass and does not rely on measuring height or weight.

Controlled Carbohydrate Meal Plan

A controlled carbohydrate meal plan (CCMP) in hospitalized PWD is one of the safest methods due to consistency from day to day but still gives the patient some flexibility on the food groups from which they can choose to meet the quantity of grams of carbohydrate allowed. Having the information on carbohydrate on the hospital menu is very helpful to the patient. The CCMP also helps with meeting glycemic goals by matching prandial insulin dose to the carbohydrate content of the meal.

Varied Meal Content and Mealtimes

Some hospitals allow patients to order food at any time. Patient satisfaction is greater with this method but carries an increased risk for missing insulin if the nurse is not notified by either the patient or food delivery service that the patient received a food tray.[9] If the patient is ordering a varied amount of carbohydrate from meal to meal and day to day, it is difficult to achieve glycemic targets if the same prandial dose is being used. Consider implementing insulin to carbohydrate ratio if the patients are eating a variable amount of carbohydrate from meal to meal and day to day.

Carbohydrate Counting

If a PWD is carbohydrate counting prior to hospitalization, then it should be continued in the hospital. The provider would write the prandial insulin orders based on 1 unit covering a certain amount of grams of carbohydrate and the nurse would assess the amount of carbohydrate the patient is consuming and calculate the insulin dose and administer the prandial insulin. If a patient uses an insulin pump, the patient enters the carbohydrate grams into the insulin pump, and the pump will calculate the amount of insulin needed and deliver the insulin dose. The nurse documents the grams consumed by the patient and the insulin pump bolus dose.[9]

NOTHING BY MOUTH STATUS, CLEAR LIQUID DIET, AND NUTRITIONAL SUPPLEMENTS

Clear and full liquid diets should provide no less than 130 g of carbohydrate per day.[3] Whitman reported that advancing slowly from clear liquid to full liquid to regular diet may possibly contribute to delayed healing and advancing from nothing by mouth (NPO) status to regular diet is generally well-tolerated. The addition of an oral nutrition supplement has been shown to reduce rehospitalization. Lower carbohydrate supplements have less impact on fasting and postprandial blood glucose.[3]

The 2023 American Society of Anesthesiologists practices guidelines for enteral nutrition (EN) and parenteral nutrition (PN).

EN and PN contributes to hyperglycemia due to increased insulin resistance, stress hormones, and decreased activity. In patients receiving PN, there is loss of the incretin effect since the gastrointestinal (GI) tract is bypassed.[10] The incretin effect is when oral glucose stimulates the release of gut hormones including glucagon-like-peptide 1 and glucose-dependent insulinotropic peptide, which stimulates glucose-dependent insulin secretion.[11] If nutrition is delivered intravenous then those hormones are not released, thus contributing to hyperglycemia. Another way to think about the incretin effect is that oral glucose elicits a higher insulin secretory response than intravenous glucose. Hyperglycemia while receiving EN and PN is associated with increased morbidity and mortality. Laesser, Cumming, Reber, and colleagues conducted a systematic literature review of glucose management of noncritically ill hospitalized patients receiving PN and/or EN and reported the following:

EN recommendations:

- Alter macronutrient distribution with the use of non-glucose sources of carbohydrate and adding fiber.
- Use of diabetes specific formulas.
- In critically ill patients, the use of a lipid-based rather than an iso-energetic glucose-based formula is preferred and reducing the carbohydrate and energy amount is helpful with managing hyperglycemia.
- Using basal insulin plus short or rapid acting insulin produces better glucose control compared to using a correctional scale only

PN recommendations:

- Adding regular insulin to the PN bag based on the carbohydrate content.

EN and total parenteral nutrition (TPN) recommendations:

- The use of intravenous insulin infusion with an algorithm provided better blood glucose control but requires intensive nursing care and is often not practical outside ICUs.[10]

ENTERAL NUTRITION IN PERSON WITH DIABETES

More than 30% of patients receiving EN experience hyperglycemia.[10] There are few studies to evaluate the impact of EN on blood glucose but elevated blood glucose while receiving enteral nutrition increases morbidity and mortality. An expert panel of 10 clinical nutrition specialists convened to address the use of EN in PWD and those with stress hyperglycemia.[12] They evaluated 2992 scenarios and divided issues into:

- The type of formula used
- Method of administration
- Infusion site

- Treatment of diabetes
- GI complications

The panel recommended in stable PWD to use a normal-calorie and protein diabetes formula and in unstable PWD to use high protein and normal calorie diabetes formula. If the patient has a pressure ulcer, then the use of a high protein normal calorie diabetes formula or a formula specific for presence of pressure ulcer is recommended. If constipation is present, they recommend the use of a formula with fiber in patients who are stable and meeting glycemic goal. If diarrhea is present, then the use of a formula with soluble fiber is recommended. If the patient has kidney disease, then that takes over all other issues and a formula specific for kidney disease is used. In PWD and obesity or pressure ulcer, protein formulas may be used. They also recommended the use of intermittent EN in outpatients, stable inpatients, especially, if constipation is present and continuous in those not stable. The preferred route of EN is gastric infusion in all patients except those with gastroparesis where post-pyloric infusion is preferred. They recommended for the treatment of hyperglycemia in PWD receiving EN.

- Metformin can be used in those less than 70 y with no comorbidities and increased cardiovascular risk, and in those over 70 y with no comorbidities with BMI over 40 and/or increased cardiovascular risk. Metformin would not be used in any PWD with poor renal and/or liver function.
- Sulfonylureas should not be used.
- Meglitinides: there was no consensus but could possibly be used for bolus tube feeding.
- Insulin therapy in those with continuous enteral nutrition.
- Basal insulin for most.
- Regular or rapid-acting insulin as a fixed bolus plus a correctional scale for treating hyperglycemia.[12] The ADA recommends 1 unit insulin per 10 to 15 g of carbohydrate in the formula.[9]

Insulin therapy in those in intermittent EN:

- Basal insulin for most.
- Rapid or ultra-rapid acting insulin as a fixed bolus plus a correctional scale for treating hyperglycemia.[9,12] The ADA recommends 1 unit insulin per 10 to 15 g of carbohydrate in the formula.[9]

TOTAL PARENTERAL NUTRITION

TPN provides calories, carbohydrate, fat, protein, electrolytes, minerals, and vitamin via central venous catheter using the femoral, subclavian, or internal jugular vein. The indication for using TPN is if there is significant impaired GI function and the patient is not able to tolerate EN. Common reasons to use TPN include:

- Intestinal obstruction and pseudo-obstruction
- Used to provide bowel rest for GI fistula
- Post-operative bowel anastomosis leak
- Severe diarrhea or vomiting causing malnutrition
- Certain hypercatabolic states
- NPO status for greater than 7 d in critically ill patients or in those with inflammatory bowel disease

Hyperglycemia is found in more than 50% of patients receiving TPN.[10] Patients with diabetes who receive TPN most likely will need insulin added to the bag to treat the dextrose in the bag. The recommendation is to start with 1 unit regular insulin for every 10 to 15 g of carbohydrate to be added to the TPN bag. If the patient has a basal insulin requirement prior to TPN, it should be continued. A correctional scale is usually ordered while determining the correct amount of insulin is needed for the TPN bag.[9]

SUMMARY

Medical nutritional therapy for people with diabetes should be individualized for PWD to meet their nutritional, weight, lipid, blood pressure, and the glycemic goals. The individual food choices should include foods the patient enjoys eating but is mainly plant based with less animal products, processed foods, and concentrated sweets. In the hospitalized PWD, malnutrition is common and nutrition screening tools should be utilized to identify PWD with malnutrition or risk of malnutrition to provide nutrition support. Malnutrition increases the risk for adverse outcomes including infection, impaired healing, longer length-of-stay, rehospitalization, morbidity, and mortality. For hospitalized and outpatient PWD, an individualized meal plan based on a nutrition assessment and patient food preferences and patient education should be carried out by a registered dietitian who is knowledgeable in assessing nutrition status and working with PWD. Meal planning in PWD is an important piece in achieving glycemic, lipid, blood pressure, and weight goals.

CLINICS CARE POINTS

- MNT should be based on the PDW's individualized nutrition requirements and food preferences, with the goal of meeting glycemic, lipid, blood pressure, and weight goals.
- A nutrition assessment and creation of an individualized meal plan should be designed by and the patient counseled by a registered dietitian knowledgeable in working with PWD.
- The nutrition method should consider patient preferences on eating patterns and type of foods as much as possible.
- Hospitalized PWD should be screened for malnutrition using a standardized tool.
- Hospitalized PWD with malnutrition or risk of malnutrition should receive nutrition support to prevent or treat nutrition.
- Hospitalized PWD who are on specialized diets including NPO status, clear or full liquid diets, pureed diets, EN and/or PN need to have the blood glucose closely monitored and diabetes medications prescribed appropriately to reduce risk of hypoglycemia and severe hyperglycemia.
- EN and PN will cause higher blood glucose levels compared to consuming food by mouth due to loss of incretin effect, increased stress response from the illness contributing to insulin resistance, and decreased activity.
- EN formulas should be chosen based on the nutritional requirements of the patient.
- Insulin dosing for EN is based on the carbohydrate content of the formula and frequency of prandial dosing depends on whether the tube feeding is continuous or bolus.
- Insulin dosing for PN is also based on the carbohydrate content in the bag and the insulin should be added to the bag rather than subcutaneous.
- Patients with a basal insulin requirement before EN and PN will still need basal insulin to maintain glycemic goals when not receiving nutrition.

- Patients with a basal insulin requirement will still need basal insulin even if the patient is not receiving any nutrition; however, the dose will probably need to be reduced if the patient is fasting for a prolonged period or overall receiving less than usual amounts of calories and carbohydrates due to decreased liver glucose production.

DISCLOSURE

The author does not have any conflicts of interest to disclose.

REFERENCES

1. American Diabetes Association. 5. Facilitating positive health behaviors and well-being to improve health outcomes: standards of care in diabetes—2024. Diabetes Care 2024;47(Supplement_1):S77–110.
2. Evert AB, Dennison M, Gardner CD, et al. Nutrition therapy for adults with diabetes or prediabetes: a consensus report. Diabetes Care 2019;42(5):731.
3. Whitham D. Nutrition management of diabetes in acute care. Can J Diabetes 2014;38(2):90–3.
4. Skytte MJ, Samkani A, Petersen AD, et al. A carbohydrate-reduced high-protein diet improves HbA 1c and liver fat content in weight stable participants with type 2 diabetes: a randomised controlled trial. Diabetologia 2019;62:2066–78.
5. Builes-Montaño CE, Ortiz-Cano NA, Ramirez-Rincón A, et al. Efficacy and safety of carbohydrate counting versus other forms of dietary advice in patients with type 1 diabetes mellitus: a systematic review and meta-analysis of randomised clinical trials. J Hum Nutr Diet 2022;35(6):1030–42.
6. Dent E, Hoogendijk E, Visvanathan R, et al. Malnutrition screening and assessment in hospitalised older people: a review. J Nutr Health Aging 2019;23(5): 431–41.
7. Yuan Z, Jiang C, Lao G, et al. Effectiveness of Global Leadership Initiative on Malnutrition and Subjective Global Assessment for diagnosing malnutrition and predicting wound healing in patients with diabetic foot ulcers. Br J Nutr 2024; 123(1):1–10.
8. House M, Gwaltney C. Malnutrition screening and diagnosis tools: implications for practice. Nutr Clin Pract 2022;37(1):12–22.
9. Committee ADAPP. 16. Diabetes care in the hospital: standards of care in diabetes—2024. Diabetes Care 2023;47(Supplement_1):S295–306.
10. Laesser CI, Cumming P, Reber E, et al. Management of glucose control in non-critically ill, hospitalized patients receiving parenteral and/or enteral nutrition: a systematic review. J Clin Med 2019;8(7):935.
11. Zhang X, Young RL, Bound M, et al. Comparative effects of proximal and distal small intestinal glucose exposure on glycemia, incretin hormone secretion, and the incretin effect in health and type 2 diabetes. Diabetes Care 2019;42(4):520–8.
12. Rebollo-Pérez MI, Florencio Ojeda L, García-Luna PP, et al. Standards for the use of enteral nutrition in patients with diabetes or stress hyperglycaemia: expert consensus. Nutrients 2023;15(23):4976.

Management of Hypertension in Patients with Diabetes

Anne Brinkman, DNP, APRN, AGNP-C

KEYWORDS

- Diabetes mellitus • Hypertension • Blood pressure • Diabetes management
- Diabetes outcomes

KEY POINTS

- The target blood pressure for patients with diabetes is less than 130/80.
- Lifestyle modification and pharmacotherapy should be used as part of an overall diabetes treatment plan.
- Diabetes patients have more severe hypertension compared to non-diabetes patients and may require more intense pharmacologic therapy.
- Reaching and maintaining blood pressure goals leads to decreased risk for death and microvascular and macrovascular complications of diabetes.

BACKGROUND: WHY BLOOD PRESSURE CONTROL IS IMPORTANT

Atherosclerotic cardiovascular disease, leading to stroke and myocardial infarction, remains the number one cause of death in people with diabetes. The Centers for Disease Control reported that in 2020, there were 1.68 million hospitalizations for heart disease and stroke among diabetes patients (71.6 per 1000 adults with diabetes).[1] Comorbid conditions such as hypertension (HTN) increase the risk for heart disease as well as renal failure and diabetes retinopathy, making HTN screening and management a top priority in diabetes patients.[2]

Hypertension is common among diabetes patients in the United States, with 71% to 80.6% having blood pressure (BP) above goal or requiring at least 1 medication to control BP.[1,3] Controlling HTN in diabetes patients has been shown to decrease the risk of death and microvascular and macrovascular complications of the disease.[2,4] Several meta-analyses of HTN trials have shown that maintaining systolic blood pressures less than 133 to 135 mm Hg reduces the risk of stroke by 17% to 31%, major

Department of Endocrine Neoplasia and Hormonal Disorders, The University of Texas MD Anderson Cancer Center, 1400 Pressler Street, Unit 1461, Houston, TX 77030, USA
E-mail address: AKBrinkman@mdanderson.org

Crit Care Nurs Clin N Am 37 (2025) 85–92
https://doi.org/10.1016/j.cnc.2024.08.002   **ccnursing.theclinics.com**
0899-5885/25/© 2024 Elsevier Inc. All rights reserved, including those for text and data mining, AI training, and similar technologies.

cardiovascular events by 14%, and all-cause mortality by 10%, with the greatest benefits seen in patients whose baseline BP was $\geq$140/90 mm Hg.[2]

The American Diabetes Association (ADA) highlights a multifaceted approach to reducing the risk for diabetes complications with a foundation of lifestyle modification and diabetes education and supported by 4 pillars: glycemic management, control of BP, lipid management, and utilization of pharmaceutical agents shown to have improved cardiovascular and renal outcomes.[2]

GUIDELINES AVAILABLE FOR HYPERTENSION MANAGEMENT

There are multiple resources available from respected diabetes organizations that provide guidance for HTN management in diabetes patients, including management of special populations such as the elderly. Additional guidelines published by cardiology organizations are also available as follows:.

- The American Diabetes Association: Standards of Care in Diabetes—2024[2]
- Treatment of Diabetes in Older Adults: An Endocrine Society Clinical Practice Guideline[5]
- American Association of Clinical Endocrinology Consensus Statement: Comprehensive Type 2 Diabetes Management Algorithm 2023 Update[4]

SCREENING AND DIAGNOSIS OF HYPERTENSION

The ADA recommends that diabetes patients have their BP evaluated during each patient encounter.[2] The criteria for diagnosing HTN in diabetes as set forth by the ADA includes the following

- Normal blood pressure: Below 120/80 mm Hg
- Early or pre-hypertension: Between 120/80 mm Hg and 130/80 mm Hg
- Hypertension: 130/80 mm Hg or higher

The American Heart Association (AHA) and American College of Cardiology (ACC) further stratify HTN into stages:[3]

- Normal blood pressure: Below 120/80 mm Hg
- Elevated blood pressure: 120 to 129/80 mm Hg
- Stage 1 hypertension: 130 to 139/80 to 89 mm Hg
- Stage 2 hypertension: $\geq$140/90 mm Hg

In contrast, to the ADA, AHA, and ACC, the 2023 European Society of Hypertension (ESH) guidelines, endorsed by the International Society of Hypertension and the European Renal Association, have a higher threshold for diagnosing hypertension, and further classify HTN into stages based on co-morbid conditions:[6]

- Optimal: less than 120/ less than 80 mm Hg
- Normal: 120 to 129/80 to 84 mm Hg
- High-normal: 130 to 139/85 to 89 mm Hg
- Grade 1 hypertension: 140 to 159/90 to 99 mm Hg
- Grade 2 hypertension: 160 to 179/100 to 109 mm Hg
- Grade 3 hypertension: $\geq$180/$\geq$110
- Stage 1: Uncomplicated hypertension (without end-organ damage or cardiovascular disease (CVD))
- Stage 2: Presence of end-organ damage or diabetes or chronic kidney disease (CKD) stage 3
- Stage 3: Established CVD or advanced CKD stage 4 or 5

Regardless of the threshold used to diagnose HTN, patients with BP readings greater than 130/80 mm Hg should have the diagnosis confirmed over 2 to 3 readings at separate visits, or through home BP monitoring.[3] However, if the BP is ≥180/110 mm Hg in a patient with known CVD, the diagnosis of HTN can be made based on a single visit and treatment should be initiated promptly.[2,3,6]

Multiple guidelines highlight the importance of accurate BP measurement. Equipment should be regularly serviced and calibrated and staff as well as patients should be trained on proper technique for BP measurement. Patients should be seated in a chair with BP measured after 5 minutes of rest. The feet should both be on the floor (legs should not be crossed) and the arm supported at the level of the heart. The BP cuff should be chosen according to the patient's size based on upper arm circumference as shown in **Fig. 1**. Finally, the patient should not talk during BP measurement.[2–4,6]

Home BP monitoring is useful in confirming and monitoring patients with a diagnosis of HTN as well as evaluating for "white coat syndrome" or "masked hypertension." White coat syndrome occurs when BP readings are only elevated in the office setting and occurs in 13% to 35% of patients. Masked HTN is when BP readings are normal in the office but elevated at home and occurs in 14% to 30% of patients.[3] In addition to confirming a suspected diagnosis, home BP monitoring can improve a patient's compliance with their HTN treatment regimen.[2]

BLOOD PRESSURE TARGETS FOR PEOPLE WITH DIABETES

Respected diabetes organizations such as the ADA, the American Association of Clinical Endocrinology, and the Endocrine Society performed extensive literature and guideline review and agree that the BP target for most diabetes patients should be less than 130/80 mm Hg, and that pharmacologic treatment is indicated if BP exceeds that threshold. Slightly lower targets may be appropriate for patients with certain risk factors, such as history of stroke or progressive kidney disease, and slightly higher targets for populations at higher risk for orthostatic hypotension and/or falls.[2,4,5] The 2017 clinical practice guidelines published by the AHA/ACC do not routinely recommend pharmacologic treatment for stage 1 HTN (BP 130–139/80–89 mm Hg), except in the setting of known atherosclerotic cardiovascular disease (ASCVD) defined as coronary disease, congestive heart failure, and stroke, or in those with a 10-year risk for ASCVD event of ≥10%. Instead, they recommended lifestyle modification and reassessment in 3 to 6 months for milder HTN in low-risk persons. The rationale for not recommending a lower target was the lack of randomized controlled trial data demonstrating significant benefits in treating BP less than 140/90 in people with low 10-year ASCVD risk scores.[3] However, they acknowledge that most persons with diabetes will inherently have an ASCVD risk score of ≥10%, therefore, their recommendation for persons with diabetes is to initiate pharmacologic therapy even in stage 1 HTN, consistent with the ADA guidelines. The AHA/ACC also later released a scientific

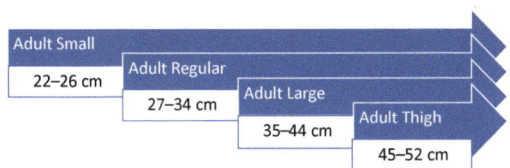

Fig. 1. Using arm circumference to choose blood pressure cuff size.

statement in support of pharmacologic therapy for stage 1 HTN, even in low-risk patients, if the goal of less than 130/80 is not reached after 6 months of lifestyle management.[7]

Targeting a BP of less than 120/80 is not recommended for most patients given the increased risk for adverse events such as orthostatic hypotension, electrolyte disturbances, and kidney injury.[2] Patients aged 65 or older are at higher risk for adverse events, and should target a BP of 140/90 mm Hg unless they belong to a higher risk group, such as those with kidney disease or history of stroke, in which case a lower BP target of 130/80 mm Hg may be considered through a shared decision-making process.[5] Pregnant women with diabetes who develop gestational HTN should be treated if the BP exceeds 140/90 mm Hg and have a target treatment range of 110 to 135/85 mm Hg.[2] Blood pressure targets based on the ADA and Endocrine Society guidelines are summarized in **Table 1**.[2,5]

TREATMENT OF HYPERTENSION

Treatment of HTN is multifaceted including.

- Lifestyle modification
- Pharmacologic therapy
- Blood pressure monitoring (discussed previously)

Treatment approaches vary based upon the BP values upon diagnosis and may range from lifestyle modification and close monitoring to the immediate initiation of more than 1 pharmacologic agent. **Table 2** summarizes the overall treatment approach based on the level of BP upon diagnosis of HTN, based on the ADA guidelines.[2]

Lifestyle Modification

Lifestyle is an important aspect of HTN and overall diabetes control. The ADA recommends several interventions for diabetes patients who have a BP greater than 120/80 mm Hg, and the recommendations are similar to those listed in the AHA/ACC and ESH guidelines for hypertensive patients.[2,3,6] The recommendations include as follows:

- Weight loss (in overweight or obese people)
- Dietary modification
- Limiting alcohol intake
- Tobacco cessation
- Physical activity/Exercise

Lifestyle modification alone may be sufficient for patients with pre-HTN or stage 1 HTN without elevated ASCVD risk. Regardless of the necessity of pharmacologic therapy, all persons will benefit from improved BP control with lifestyle modification, and those requiring pharmacologic therapy may be able to reduce the number of

Table 1 Blood pressure targets recommended by endocrine experts	
Group	Blood Pressure Target
Most adults with diabetes	<130/80 mm Hg
Elderly, frail, or high risk for falls	<140–160/80–90 mm Hg
Pregnant individuals with diabetes	110–135/85 mm Hg

Table 2
Initial recommendations for management of hypertension based on blood pressure reading

Blood Pressure	Intervention
Pre-hypertension (120/80–129/79)	Lifestyle interventions (weight loss, diet, exercise, alcohol reduction, and smoking cessation)
Hypertension (≥130/80)	Lifestyle interventions + 1 pharmacologic agent + re-evaluation in 1 mo
Severe hypertension (>150/90)	Lifestyle interventions + 2 pharmacologic agents + re-evaluation in no later than 1 mo

medications through lifestyle modification.[6] The expected improvements in BP based on lifestyle intervention in persons with HTN are shown in **Table 3**.[2,3,6] Dietary modification is one of the most effective lifestyle modifications, with the Dietary Approaches to Stop Hypertension (DASH) diet being a cornerstone recommendation for patients with HTN.[2–4,6] The DASH diet encourages intake of vegetables, fruits, and whole grains while limiting high-sugar and high-fat foods. Salt intake reduction is also a key feature of the DASH diet.[2,6] Stress reduction techniques such as yoga, mindfulness, and meditation also have beneficial effects on blood pressure management, and internet or mobile applications can help improve compliance with lifestyle interventions as well as pharmacologic therapies.[2]

Choice of Pharmacologic Therapy

Diabetes patients often have more severe hypertension than non-diabetes patients and require more than 1 medication to control BP in most cases.[5] In patients whose BP is ≥150/90 mm Hg, 2 medications, or a combination medication should be considered as initial therapy.[2–6] **Fig. 2** summarizes the initial treatment approach recommended by the ADA based on the presence of diabetes kidney disease (DKD), coronary artery disease (CAD), and the BP at diagnosis.[2]

First-line pharmacologic therapy for most diabetes patients, including patients 65 and older, should include an angiotensin-converting enzyme inhibitor (ACEis) or angiotensin II receptor blocker (ARBs) because these agents are efficacious, well tolerated, slow progression of DKD, and reduce the risk of heart disease.[2,4,5] In patients without

Table 3
Expected blood pressure reductions with lifestyle modification

Lifestyle Intervention	Recommendation	Expected Reduction in Blood Pressure
Weight Loss	Reach ideal weight or at least ≥5% weight loss, ideally 10%–15%	−1 mm Hg per 1 kg lost up to 6.5 mm Hg
Dietary Modification	Dietary Approaches to Stop Hypertension Diet including reducing sodium (<1500–2300 mg/day) and increasing potassium; Mediterranean diet	−4.8–11 mm Hg
Physical Activity	90–150 min of moderate intensity aerobic exercise weekly	−5 to 8 mm Hg
Limiting Alcohol Intake	≤2 servings per day for Men ≤1 serving per day for Women	−3–5 mm Hg

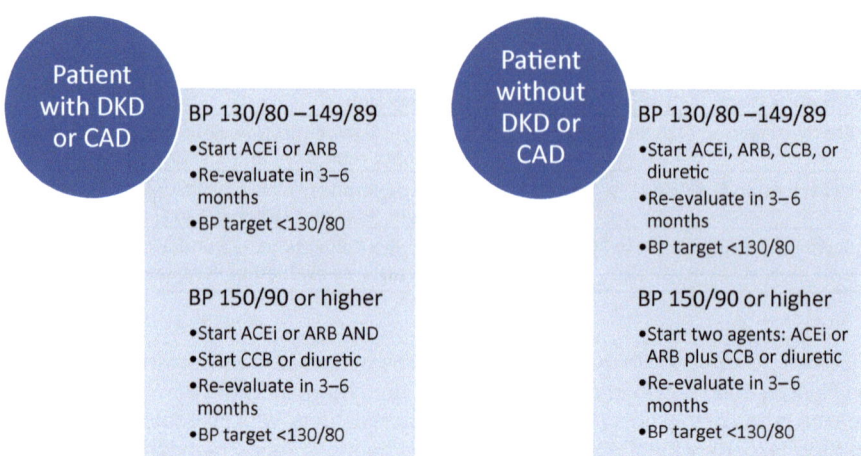

Fig. 2. American Diabetes Association approach to starting pharmacologic therapy in diabetes.

DKD or CAD, dihydropyridine calcium channel blockers or thiazide-like diuretics are alternative first-line agents. Clinicians should monitor serum creatinine, estimated glomerular filtration rate, and potassium levels 1 to 2 weeks after initiation of pharmacologic agents, and at least annually thereafter.[2]

In patients whose BP remains uncontrolled despite the use of the 3 first-line drug classes (ACEi or ARB, calcium channel blocker, and diuretic), second-line treatment with a mineralocorticoid receptor antagonist can be considered, however, clinicians should be aware of the risk for more significant hyperkalemia when adding these agents to ACEi or ARB therapy.[2] Beta blockers may also be considered and can decrease mortality in patients who have already suffered a myocardial infarction,

Table 4
Cautious prescribing of anti-hypertensives

Pharmaceutical Class	Contraindications/Cautions
Angiotensin-converting enzyme inhibitors/angiotensin II receptor blockers	Pregnancy, history of angioedema, hyperkalemia, renal artery stenosis Women of childbearing potential
Calcium Channel Blockers	Dihydropyridine: Tachycardia, heart failure, lower extremity edema Non-Dihydropyridine: Arrhythmias, heart failure, other medications sensitive to cytochrome P450 3A4 (CYP3A4)
Thiazide diuretics	Hyponatremia, sulfa allergy, urinary obstruction, hypercalcemia, hypokalemia
Beta-blocker	Severe asthma, AV-block, bradycardia, asthma, athletes
Mineralocorticoid Receptor Antagonists	Hyperkalemia, advanced CKD, other medications sensitive to CYP3A4

Adapted from 2023 ESH Guidelines for the management of arterial hypertension Mancia, G., Kreutz, R., Brunstrom, M., Burnier, M., Grassi, G., Januszewicz, A., . . . Kjeldsen, S. E. (2023). 2023 ESH Guidelines for the management of arterial hypertension. *Journal of Hypertension, 41*(12), 1874-2071. https://doi.org/10.1097/HJH.0000000000003480.

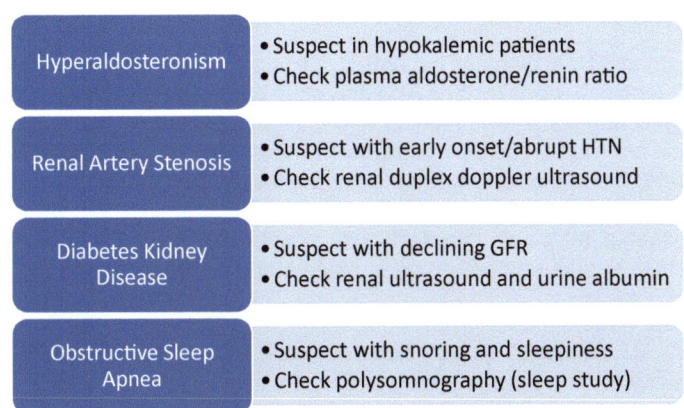

Hyperaldosteronism	• Suspect in hypokalemic patients • Check plasma aldosterone/renin ratio
Renal Artery Stenosis	• Suspect with early onset/abrupt HTN • Check renal duplex doppler ultrasound
Diabetes Kidney Disease	• Suspect with declining GFR • Check renal ultrasound and urine albumin
Obstructive Sleep Apnea	• Suspect with snoring and sleepiness • Check polysomnography (sleep study)

Fig. 3. Causes of secondary hypertension.

have angina, or heart failure. Women of childbearing potential should be counseled that treatment with ACEi, ARB, and spironolactone are contraindicated during pregnancy as they may cause birth defects.[2] Women who are pregnant or plan to become pregnant may be treated with methyldopa, labetalol, nifedipine, or hydralazine. Additional safety considerations in choice of blood pressure agent are shown in **Table 4**.[6]

Additional pharmacologic agents such as clonidine, hydralazine, or alpha 1 receptor antagonists may be added when BP remains above goal. However, patients with refractory HTN despite at least 3 pharmacologic agents, or with suspicious clinical findings, should be evaluated for secondary HTN related to hyperaldosteronism, renal artery stenosis, diabetes kidney disease, or obstructive sleep apnea (**Fig. 3**).[2,3,6] Additional, less common causes of secondary HTN, such as hormonal disorders, should also be considered based on physical examination and clinical history, and referral to an HTN specialist should be considered.[2]

BLOOD PRESSURE MANAGEMENT IN ACUTE CARE

Patients presenting to the emergency or otherwise admitted for acute care may have pre-existing HTN diagnoses that need to be managed or may be experiencing hypertensive urgency or emergency during a hospital admission for another reason. Patients should be educated on medications that can increase blood pressure (**Box 1**).[3] Hypertensive emergencies include severe HTN associated with stroke, acute cardiac conditions, acute kidney failure, drug overdose-related HTN, pheochromocytomas, and severe pre-eclampsia. These patients should be admitted for rapid treatment with intravenous medication. Hypertensive urgency is severe hypertensive, but without acute organ damage, and these patients may be able to be treated conservatively with oral medications.[6]

Box 1
Medications and supplements that increase blood pressure

Medication/Supplement
  Nonsteroidal anti-inflammatory drugs, acetaminophen, estrogens, steroids, antidepressants, nasal decongestants, stimulants, substance abuse, licorice, ephedra, St. John's Wort, yohimbine, high-dose ginseng, ma huang, diet pills

---

SUMMARY

Management of HTN in diabetes patients is critical to preventing complications of diabetes and increased mortality. The ADA and other respected guidelines recommend a multi-pronged approach to screening and initiating treatment, highlighting lifestyle modification and pharmacologic therapy. The target BP for most patients with diabetes is 130/80, and maintaining this target decreases the risk for stroke, cardiovascular events, and end-organ damage. Critical care nurses should be aware that HTN in diabetes patients is typically more difficult to control compared to non-diabetes patients and may require multiple drugs to reach blood pressure targets.

CLINICS CARE POINTS

- HTN is present in 71% to 80.6% of diabetes patients in the United States.
- Lifestyle modification alone may be effective in mild hypertension or pre-hypertension.
- The ADA recommends starting pharmacologic therapy when BP is $\geq$130/80.
- Initiate pharmacologic treatment with 2 drugs if BP is $\geq$150/90.
- Use ACEi or ARB as first-line drugs for HTN.
- Consider causes of secondary HTN in patients requiring 3 or more drugs to control BP.
- Follow up with patients monthly until BP targets are reached.

DISCLOSURE

There are no commercial or financial conflicts of interest.

REFERENCES

1. Centers for Disease Control and Prevention, National diabetes statistics report website, Available at: https://www.cdc.gov/diabetes/php/data-research/index.html, (Accessed 14 July 2024), 2024.
2. American Diabetes Association. Cardiovascular disease and risk management: Standards of care in diabetes- 2024. Diabetes Care 2024;47:S179–218.
3. Whelton PK, Carey RM, Aronow WS, et al. 2017 ACC/AHA/AAPA/ABC/ACPM/AGS/APhA/ASH/ASPC/NMA/PCNA guideline for the prevention, detection, evaluation, and management of high blood pressure in adults: a report of the American College of Cardiology/American Heart Association Task Force. Hypertension 2018;(71):e13–115.
4. Samson SL, Vellanki P, Blonde L, et al. American Association of Clinical Endocrinology Consensus Statement: comprehensive type 2 diabetes management algorithm–2023 update. Endocr Pract 2023;29(5):305–40.
5. LeRoith D, Biessels GJ, Braithwaite SS, et al. Treatment of diabetes in older adults: an endocrine society clinical practice guideline. J Clin Endocrinol Metab 2019;104(5):1520–74.
6. Mancia G, Kreutz R, Brunstrom M, et al. 2023 ESH guidelines for the management of arterial hypertension. J Hypertens 2023;41(12):1874–2071.
7. Jones DW, Whelton PK, Allen N, et al. Management of stage 1 hypertension in adults with a low 10-year risk for cardiovascular disease: filling a guidance gap: a scientific statement from the American Heart Association. Hypertension 2021;(77):e58–67.

Management of Immunotherapy-Induced Type 1 Diabetes

Veronica Brady, PhD, MSN, BSN[a,b,*]

KEYWORDS

- Immunotherapy • Checkpoint inhibitors • Type 1 diabetes • Hyperglycemia
- Diabetic ketoacidosis • Insulin

KEY POINTS

- Blood glucose should be monitored before, during, and after exposure to immunotherapy.
- People with sudden onset of hyperglycemia following treatment with immune checkpoint inhibitors should have c-peptide/random blood glucose obtained to assess insulin production.
- People diagnosed with immunotherapy-induced type 1 diabetes will require insulin for the rest of their lives.

INTRODUCTION

Immunotherapy has been used to treat a wide range of health conditions from allergic reactions to organ transplants to infectious diseases to cancer. As with most drugs, immunotherapy agents are not without side effects. These immune-related adverse effects impact various organ systems including dermatology, pulmonary, gastrointestinal, endocrine, cardiovascular, neurologic, and musculoskeletal.[1] However, the most notable and widely discussed side effects are those related to immunotherapy also known as immune checkpoint inhibitors (ICIs). In 2013, ICIs were described as the "breakthrough treatment of the year."[2] Endocrinopathies are the most common adverse effects associated with ICIs. The organs most commonly affected are the pancreas, thyroid, adrenal glands, and pituitary. One of the life-threatening adverse effects associated with ICIs is the rapid destruction of β cells in the pancreas leading to type 1 diabetes (T1D). While rare, this adverse effect has life-changing implications.

[a] Department of Research, University of Texas Health- Cizik School of Nursing, 6901 Bertner Avenue, Suite 567E, Houston, TX, USA; [b] The University of Texas MD Anderson Cancer Center, 1515 Holcombe Boulevard, Houston, TX 77030, USA
* Corresponding author. 6901 Bertner Avenue, Suite 567E, Houston, TX.
E-mail addresses: Veronica.j.brady@uth.tmc.edu; vbrady@mdanderson.org; vrnca1@hotmail.com

Crit Care Nurs Clin N Am 37 (2025) 93–102
https://doi.org/10.1016/j.cnc.2024.07.002   **ccnursing.theclinics.com**
0899-5885/25/© 2024 Elsevier Inc. All rights are reserved, including those for text and data mining, AI training, and similar technologies.

IMMUNE CHECKPOINT INHIBITORS DEFINED

Immunotherapy has become an established agent for the treatment of malignancy, with the most widely used method being the administration of monoclonal antibodies against immune checkpoint molecules that inhibit T-cell activation.[3] The drugs are thought to "release the immune brakes" leading to regression of cancer.[4] Immunotherapy involves drugs that block immune checkpoints allowing the body's immune cells to respond more strongly to cancer cells. Immunotherapy is a "living drug"; thus, adverse effects can occur weeks to years after the drug was last administered.[2]

CLASSES OF IMMUNE CHECKPOINT INHIBITOR DRUGS AND IMMUNE CHECKPOINT INHIBITOR-INDUCED TYPE 1 DIABETES

There are 3 classes of ICI agents: cytotoxic T-lymphocyte antigen 4 (CTLA-4) blocking antibody CTLA-4i, anti-programed cell death protein 1 (PD-1), and anti-programed cell death protein ligand 1 (PD-L1). The first ICI agent approved by the Federal Drug Administration, for the treatment of advanced melanoma, was ipilumumab in 2010. Since that time, 6 additional ICI agents have been approved (**Table 1**).

ICIs have been linked to new-onset insulin-dependent diabetes mellitus or immune checkpoint inhibitor-associated T1D (ICI-T1D). The drug most commonly associated with ICI-T1D is ipilumumab (**Table 2**). However, overtime these drugs are more often used in combination; thus, the prevalence of ICI-TID has increased. People who develop ICI-T1D often present with severe hyperglycemia or diabetic ketoacidosis (DKA). ICI-T1D appears to occur more abruptly than autoimmune T1D, and there are several differences in the characteristics of these diseases (**Table 3**). ICI-T1D has a rapid onset and was initially thought to be more common among minorities (Asian, Black) and older adults. However, recent studies have reported no difference in race and the adverse effects of ICIs can occur at any age.[5,6]

PATIENT PRESENTATION

Patients with ICI-T1D may present in different ways due to worsening type 2 diabetes or new onset T1D. Approximately 2 out of 3 of patients will present in DKA, while others will have profound hyperglycemia. The usual presenting symptoms are polyuria, polydipsia, polyphagia, weight loss, dehydration, and lethargy[11] (**Fig. 1**).

Depending on the onset of the severity of symptoms, patients may start insulin therapy as an outpatient. Most often these patients present in distress in an acute care setting. The diagnosis of DKA is made based on the following: blood glucose (BG) greater than 250 mg/dL, pH less than 7.3, serum bicarbonate less than 18mEq/L, beta-hydroxybutyrate (B-ohb) greater than 3, elevated anion gap (AG), positive urine ketones, and dehydration. Once the diagnosis is made, treatment with insulin is essential.

Keep in mind that *not* all patients who present in DKA have T1D, ICI induced, or otherwise. The diagnosis of ICI-T1D is made based on the criteria listed in **Box 1**.

ACUTE TREATMENT OF IMMUNE CHECKPOINT INHIBITOR-INDUCED TYPE 1 DIABETES

Patients presenting with DKA will require insulin treatment via infusion. In most hospital settings, patients requiring insulin infusion/drip are treated in the intensive care unit (ICU). Most insulin drip protocols are standard, requiring the use of 0.9NS intravenous fluid (IVF), an insulin infusion (regular insulin), and hourly BG monitoring. Changes in IVF and insulin drip rates are based on BG readings. Treatment with insulin drip usually

Table 1
Immunotherapy drugs

Year of FDA Approval	Drug	Mechanism of Action	Diseases Treated
2016	Atezolizumab	Binds to PDL-1 selectively preventing the interaction between PD-1 and B7.1 receptors on T cells	NSCLC, SCLC Basal cell carcinoma Melanoma Urothelial carcinoma Hepatocellular carcinoma
2018	Cemiplimab	Binds to PD-1 and blocks its interactions with the ligands PD-L1 and PD-L2, releases PD-1 pathway-mediated inhibition of immune responses	Cutaneous small cell carcinoma Basal cell carcinoma NSCLC
2016	Durvalumab	It blocks the interaction between PD-L1 and PD-1 as well as CD80 (B7.1) on T cells and enhances antitumor immune responses, allowing T cells to kill tumor cells	Urothelial carcinoma NSCLC, SCLC
2015	Nivolumab	Engineered IgG4 monoclonal antibody Regulates T-cell activation by blocking PD-1	Advanced melanoma Esophageal urothelial carcinoma SCC, HCC, HL, HNSCC, NSCLC, RCC
2016	Pembrolizumab	Engineered IgG4 monoclonal antibody Regulates T cell activation by blocking PD-1	Advanced melanoma Cervical cancer Endometrial cancer Esophageal carcinoma Gastric carcinoma Mesothelioma Large B-cell lymphoma Hodgkin lymphoma Breast cancer MSI-high/MMR-deficient/TMB-high cancers NSCLC, CRC, SCC, HCC, HNSCC, RCC, CSCC, SCLC, MCC
2017	Avelumab	Binds to PD-L1 inhibiting its interaction with the PD-1 receptor prevents the inhibition of CD8+ T cells	Renal cell cancer Merkel cell carcinoma Urothelial carcinoma
2010	Ipilumumab	Expressed on the surface of activated T cells. Blocks cytotoxic T-lymphocyte antigen-4. Inhibits T-cell-mediated response	Advance melanoma Renal cell cancer Hepatocellular cancer NSCLC Colorectal cancer mesothelioma

Abbreviations: BC, breast cancer; BCC, basal cell carcinoma; CRC, colorectal cancer; CSCC, cutaneous squamous cell carcinoma; HCC, hepatocellular carcinoma; HL, Hodgkin lymphoma; HNSCC, head and neck squamous cell carcinoma; MCC, Merkel cell carcinoma; MMR, mismatch repair; MSI, microsatellite instability; NSCLC, non-small cell lung cancer; RCC, renal cell carcinoma; SCC, squamous cell carcinoma; SCLC, small cell lung cancer; TMB, tumor mutational burden.

Table 2
Immunotherapy drugs associated with type 1 diabetes

Drug	Associated Prevalence of Diabetes	Nursing Considerations
Checkpoint inhibitors		
PD-1 Atezolizumab (Tecentriq®)	Type 1 diabetes mellitus: 0.3%	For grade 3–4 endocrinopathies: Withhold until clinically stable or permanently discontinue depending on severity (Genentech, Inc, 2021).
Cemiplimab-rwlc (Libtayo®)	Type 1 diabetes mellitus: 0.1%	Type 1 diabetes mellitus can present with diabetic ketoacidosis. Monitor for signs and symptoms of diabetes (Regeneron Pharmaceuticals, Inc., 2021).
Durvalumab (Imfinzi®)	Type 1 diabetes mellitus: <0.1%	Type 1 diabetes mellitus can present with diabetic ketoacidosis. Monitor for signs and symptoms of diabetes. For grade 3–4 endocrinopathies: Withhold until clinically stable or permanently discontinue depending on severity (AstraZeneca Pharmaceuticals LP, 2021).
Nivolumab (Opdivo®)	Diabetes: 0.9%	Monitor for hyperglycemia or other signs and symptoms of diabetes. Initiate treatment
Pembrolizumab (Keytruda®)	Hyperglycemia: 45% Type 1 diabetes mellitus: 0.2%	Type 1 diabetes mellitus: Administer insulin. For severe hyperglycemia, withhold pembrolizumab, and administer antihyperglycemic. May resume once toxicity recovers to grade 0 or 1 (Merck & Co., Inc., 2021).
Checkpoint inhibitors		
PD-L1 Avelumab (Bavencio®)	Type 1 diabetes mellitus: 0.1%	For grade 3 or 4 endocrinopathies, withhold avelumab, and initiate appropriate medical management of toxicity. May resume avelumab after resolution of grade 0–1 and corticosteroid taper. For persistent grade 2–3 immune-mediated toxicity (lasting 12 wk or longer), permanently discontinue avelumab (EMD Serono, Inc., 2020).

(continued on next page)

Table 2
(continued)

Drug	Associated Prevalence of Diabetes	Nursing Considerations
Cytotoxic T-lymphocyte antigen-4 blocking antibody		
Ipilumumab (Yervoy®)	Diabetes occurred in 2.7%	Advise patients to contact their health care provider immediately for signs or symptoms of diabetes mellitus. For grade 3–4 endocrinopathies: Withhold until clinically stable or permanently discontinue depending on severity (Bristol-Myers Squibb Company, 2021).

continues until the patient is stabilized and the AG has closed. After the AG has closed, is it important to continue to monitor patients to ensure that DKA has completely resolved (**Box 2**). Then steps are made to transition the patient to subcutaneous insulin using multiple daily injections (MDIs).

*Note: Dietary intake destabilizes insulin drip.

Table 3
Comparison between immunotherapy type 1 diabetes and autoimmune type 1 diabetes

Characteristic	Immune Checkpoint Inhibitor-induced Type 1 Diabetes	Autoimmune Type 1 Diabetes
Pathogenesis	Occurs as an adverse event related to receiving ICI for cancer treatment Destruction of β cells by autoreactive T cells	Inappropriate autoimmune response to autoreactive T cells
Risk Factors	Use of dual CTLA-4 and PD-1/PD-L1 Preexisting non-T1DM	Environmental triggers Genetic predisposition
Age	Any age	(usually) youth
B-cell destruction	Rapid onset-faster than autoimmune—sometimes within days of ICI treatment	
Pancreas size	Pancreatic atrophy has been observed radiographically	No change in size
Prevalence of DKA	40%–76%	40.6%
Autoantibodies	Rate is lower GAD+ 5%–57%	+GAD65, IA-2 and insulin antibodies often present
HLA-DR4	Approximately 60%	50%
Impact on survival	Does not significantly impact cancer survival Long-term management of T1DM required	Long-term management of T1DM essential

Data from Refs.[7–13]

Hyperglycemia→DKA

Increased thirst, increased urination, increased hunger, blurred vision, drowsiness	Nausea and vomiting, abdominal pain, decreased appetite weakness and fatigue, mood changes, confusion, hot dry skin, hyperventilation, fruity breath

Fig. 1. Signs and symptoms of hyperglycemia versus diabetic ketoacidosis.

TRANSITIONING FROM INSULIN DRIP

There are several ways to transition patients from insulin drip to MDIs.

- *Option 1*: If the patient was on basal insulin only before admission, start the home dose of basal insulin and initiate prandial insulin in 3 divided doses with meals. Basal and prandial insulin should be balanced at 50% each. For example, if the patient requires 15 units of basal insulin, add 15 units of prandial insulin (5 units with meals 3 times a day) for a total daily dose (TDD) of 30 units.
- *Options 2:* Calculate the amount of insulin that the patient has required in the last 8 hours on the insulin drip (eg, 3 units/hour x 8 hours = 24 units) and divide this by 2 (24/2 = 12). The patient's insulin doses would be 12 units basal and 4 units prandial 3 times a day with meals = 24 units TDD.
- *Option 3:* Calculate the insulin dose using a TDD of 0.4 units/kg/day (may be as high as 1.0 units/kg/day if the patient of higher weight). For example, patient is 100 kg x 0.4 units = 40 units TDD. Basal insulin will be 20 units daily and prandial insulin will be 7 units 3 times a day with meals 41 units TDD.

Often the general rule is to start with whichever dose is lower to avoid hypoglycemia. Once the dose of basal insulin is determined, it should be given *2 hours prior to the insulin drip being discontinued.*

LONG-TERM TREATMENT OF IMMUNE CHECKPOINT INHIBITOR-INDUCED TYPE 1 DIABETES

ICI-T1D is treated the same as autoimmune T1D. In both cases, the patient has an absolute insulin deficiency due to β-cell destruction. This means that not only does the patient not produce insulin but he/she also has no protection against hypoglycemia. Therefore, while they must learn insulin administration techniques, they must also learn how to recognize and treat hypoglycemia.

INSULIN THERAPY

For people with T1D, insulin therapy should consist of long acting (basal) and short acting (bolus/prandial) in divided doses to mimic physiologic insulin production

---

Box 1
Immune checkpoint inhibitor-induced type 1 diabetes diagnosis

Criteria for diagnosis of ICI-T1D
- Previous treatment with ICI therapy
- New-onset hyperglycemia
- Low c-peptide (<0.4 ng/mL) (w/elevated BG) or presence of DKA (without prior use of sodium–glucose cotransporter 2 inhibitors)

Box 2
Steps for monitoring after diabetic ketoacidosis

1. Monitor daily electrolytes (specifically bicarbonate) in these patients for trends in the wrong direction (even if not abnormal).

2. If glycemic control is not optimal after transitioning to MDIs, check serum B-ohb to monitor for ketosis. *Sometimes B-ohb may be elevated before we see metabolic acidosis and allow for early intervention!*

3. Interpretation of B-ohb levels:
    i. Serum B-ohb less than 0.28 mmol/L suggests no evidence of ketosis
    ii. *Serum B-ohb between 0.3 and 2.9*: patient (pt) has evidence of ketone production. Recommend IV hydration and close monitoring of blood sugars with appropriate insulin treatment to avoid DKA.
    iii. *Serum B-ohb greater than 3*: concerning for DKA and requires immediate intervention.

4. Consider point of care glucose (POC) check every 4 hours overnight in patients who have had poor glycemic control during the day (at least 2 glucose values more than 200 mg/dL).

(**Fig. 2**). There are several different types of basal/bolus insulin available (**Table 4**). The regimen should be personalized for each patient based on cost, personal preferences, visual acuity, manual dexterity, and so forth (see transitioning from insulin drip for guidance on insulin doses).

Hypoglycemia

One of the pitfalls of insulin treatment is hypoglycemia. In the case of patients with ICI-T1D, hypoglycemia can occur as a result of too much insulin, missed meals, or less than anticipated dietary intake. The diagnosis of hypoglycemia is made based on the presence of 3 elements known as Whipple's triad (**Box 3**). The symptoms of hypoglycemia may range from moderate to severe based on the level of hypoglycemia (**Table 5**).

TREATMENT OF HYPOGLYCEMIA

Treatment of hypoglycemia is generally treated based on the rule of 15. The rule of 15 posits that 15 g of carbohydrate will raise BG 15 mg/dL and BG should be rechecked after 15 minutes. In the acute care setting, D50 W either ½ amp (12.5 g of carbohydrate) or a full amp (25 g of carbohydrate) is usually used to treat hypoglycemia (BG < 70 mg/dL) if the patient is not eating. Glucagon, either ready to inject or intranasal, can also be used if the patient is unable to swallow or unresponsive. In other areas of

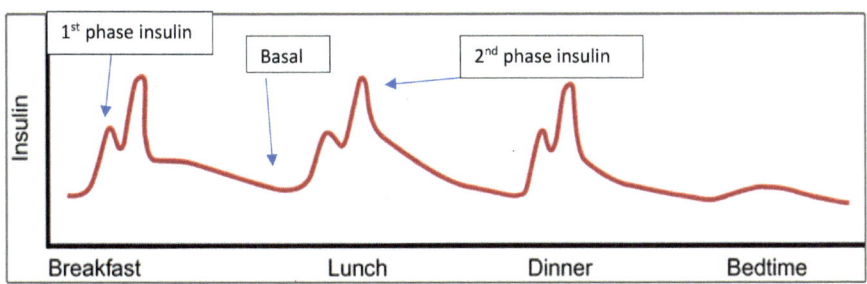

Fig. 2. Normal insulin secretion.

Table 4
Basal and bolus insulin used in the treatment of immune checkpoint inhibitor-induced type 1 diabetes

Generic Name	Brand Name	Onset	Peak	Duration
Ultrarapid-acting insulin				
Insulin Human Inhalation Powder	Afrezza	1 min	30–40 min	1.5–2 h
Aspart	Fiasp	2 min	30–60 min	3–5 h
Insulin lispro-aabc	Lyumjev/Lyumjev U-200	5–15 min	60 min	6 h
Rapid-acting insulin				
Glulisine	Apidra	5–20 min	1–3 h	3–5 h
Lispro	Humalog/Humalog U-200/ Admelog	10–20 min	1–3 h	3–5
Aspart	Novolog	10–20 min	1–3 h	3–5 h
Short-acting insulin				
Regular	Humulin R, Novolin R, Relion R	30–60 min	2–4 h	5–8 h
Regular U-500	Humulin R U-500	2.5 h	4–8 h	13–24 h
Intermediate-acting insulin				
Neutral protamine hagedorn	Humulin N, Novolin N, Relion N	1–2 h	4–12 h	14–24 h
Long-acting insulin				
Detemir	Levemir	1 h	3–14 h	Up to 24 h
Glargine U-100	Lantus/Basaglar	3–4 h	Peakless	Up to 24 h
Glargine U-300	Toujeo	6 h	Peakless	Up to 36 h
Degludec U-100/U-200	Tresiba U-100/U-200	2 h	Peakless	Up to 42 h

Box 3
Whipple's triad

1. Symptoms of low blood glucose
2. Documented plasma blood glucose less than 55 mg/dL and
3. Resolution of symptoms after blood glucose is raised.

Table 5
Levels of hypoglycemia

Level	Blood Glucose Value	Symptoms
Level 1 (mild)	<70 and ≥ 54 mg/dL	Shaking, sweating, rapid heartbeat, increased hunger (suggest a need for carbohydrate intake)
Level 2 (moderate)	<54 mg/dL	Confusion, irritability (associated with cognitive impairment and mortality)
Level 3 (severe)		Unable to function due to physical or mental changes due to low BG (requires emergency treatment → use of glucagon)

Table 6
Food and beverage containing 15 g of carbohydrate

Food/Beverage	Amount
Orange juice	4 oz
Lifesavers	5
Smarties	1 pk
Skittles	15 (fun size bag)
Honey straws	2
Glucose tablets	4–6
Jelly Beans	6 large

the hospital, or as an outpatient, if the patient is eating, hypoglycemia can be treated with food or beverage containing carbohydrates (**Table 6**).

SUMMARY

Although rare (<4%), ICI-T1D is a severe adverse effect of treatment with ICIs. Knowing that this adverse effect can happen days to years after treatment with ICI therapy makes it necessary for nurses (providers) to not only recognize those at risk for ICI-T1D but also recognize the symptoms of hyperglycemia/DKA and initiate treatment as quickly as possible. It is also important that patients who develop ICI-T1D understand that they will require insulin therapy for the rest of their lives.

CLINICS CARE POINTS

- Immunotherapy is a "living drug"; the adaptive immune response may persist for years—thus, adverse effects may be seen months after therapy is discontinued.[2]
- ICI-related symptoms often mimic symptoms of malignancy, making evaluation before initiation of treatment imperative.[2]
- Assessment for ICI-T1D should always include c-peptide with concomitant BG.
- Patients treated with immunotherapy should always carry an immunotherapy wallet card https://www.ons.org/sites/default/files/2019-01/IO Card 1-sided_Vertical.pdf.[14]

DISCLOSURE

The author is a president-elect for the Association of Diabetes Care and Education Specialist.

REFERENCES

1. Puzanov I, Diab A, Abdallah K, et al, Society for immunotherapy of cancer Toxicity management Working, Group. managing toxicities associated with immune checkpoint inhibitors: consensus recommendations from the Society for immunotherapy of cancer (SITC) Toxicity management Working Group. J Immunother Cancer 2017;5(1):95.
2. Deligiorgi MV, Panayiotidis MI, Trafalis DT. Endocrine adverse events related with immune checkpoint inhibitors: an update for clinicians. Immunotherapy 2020; 12(7):481–510.

3. Fessas P, Possamai LA, Clark J, et al. Immunotoxicity from checkpoint inhibitor therapy: clinical features and underlying mechanisms. Immunology 2020; 159(2):167–77.

4. Vaddepally RK, Kharel P, Pandey R, et al. Review of Indications of FDA-approved immune checkpoint inhibitors per NCCN Guidelines with the level of evidence. Cancers 2020;12(3). https://doi.org/10.3390/cancers12030738.

5. Chen X, Affinati AH, Lee Y, et al. Immune checkpoint inhibitors and risk of type 1 diabetes. Diabetes Care 2022;45(5):1170–6.

6. Cho YK, Jung CH. Immune-checkpoint inhibitors-induced type 1 diabetes mellitus: from its molecular mechanisms to clinical Practice. Diabetes Metab J 2023; 47(6):757–66.

7. Bagchi S, Yuan R, Engleman EG. Immune checkpoint inhibitors for the treatment of cancer: clinical impact and mechanisms of response and resistance. Annu Rev Pathol 2021;16:223–49.

8. Jensen ET, Stafford JM, Saydah S, et al. Increase in prevalence of diabetic ketoacidosis at diagnosis among Youth with type 1 diabetes: the SEARCH for diabetes in youth study. Diabetes Care 2021;44(7):1573–8.

9. Jeun R, Iyer PC, Best C, et al. Clinical outcomes of immune checkpoint inhibitor diabetes mellitus at a comprehensive cancer center. Immunotherapy 2023;15(6): 417–28.

10. Wang G, Wang J, Dong S, et al. Immune checkpoint inhibitor-associated diabetes mellitus in patients with HCC: Report of three cases and literature review. Exp Ther Med 2024;27(5):198.

11. Zhang R, Cai XL, Liu L, et al. Type 1 diabetes induced by immune checkpoint inhibitors. Chin Med J (Engl) 2020;133(21):2595–8.

12. Wright JJ, Powers AC, Johnson DB. Endocrine toxicities of immune checkpoint inhibitors. Nature Reviews 2021. https://doi.org/10.1038/s41574.021.00484.3.

13. Hattersley R, Nana M, Lansdown AJ. Endocrine complications of immunotherapies: a review. Clin Med 2021;21(2):e212–22.

14. Brady VJ. Endocrine Toxicities. In: Olsen M, LeFebvre KB, Walker SL, Dunphy EP, editors. Chemotherapy and Immunotherapy Guidelines and Recommendations for Practie. 2nd Ed. Pittsburgh, PA: Oncology Nursing Society; 2023. p. 685–99.

Hypoglycemia in Hospitalized Patients with Diabetes

Elaine Maduzia, MSN, MHA, RN, CPHQ[a],*,
Veronica Sanchez, BSN, RN, SCRN[b]

KEYWORDS

- Hypoglycemia • Inpatient • Hospital • Intensive care • Treatment • Diabetes
- Mellitus

KEY POINTS

- Hospitalized patients with diabetes can experience hypoglycemia suddenly.
- Standard of care dictates prompt treatment of hypoglycemia.
- Critically ill patients in the hospital face challenges in treating hypoglycemia management.
- Severe hypoglycemia can cause mortality.
- The prevention of hypoglycemia in the critical care setting is empirical to diabetes management.

INTRODUCTION

According to the American Diabetes Association, 1.4 million people will be diagnosed in 2024.[1] Currently, 1 out of 4 persons in the United States has diabetes mellitus but is not aware of the disease. According to Diabetes 2030, there will be a significant increase of patients with diabetes to 30% of all Americans, with a 51% increase in older adults.[2] New screening guidelines, effective in 2015, from the US Preventative Services Task Force, recommend that all adults with obesity between the ages of 40 and 70 years be screened. In 2017, diabetes was the seventh leading cause of death, specifically with diabetes documented on the death certificates.[1,3] Health care costs are increasing rapidly, by 2030 global costs are estimated at US$2.1 to 2.5 trillion. In the United States, in 2017, the total estimated cost of treating diabetes was US$414 billion, which represented 24% of total health care spending. In 2016, in the United

[a] Nurse Navigator Diabetes, Quality Department, The Woodlands Hospital, 6th Floor, Room 6702, The Woodlands, TX 77385, USA; [b] Intensive Care Unit, The Woodlands Hospital, 2nd Floor, The Woodlands, TX 77385, USA
* Corresponding author. Houston Methodist The Woodlands hospital, 17201 Interstate 45 South, The Woodlands, TX 77385.
E-mail address: emaduzia@houstonmethodist.org

Crit Care Nurs Clin N Am 37 (2025) 103–115
https://doi.org/10.1016/j.cnc.2024.09.001
0899-5885/25/© 2024 Elsevier Inc. All rights reserved, including those for text and data mining, AI training, and similar technologies.
ccnursing.theclinics.com

States, patients with diabetes were hospitalized over 7.8 billion times.[3] In lieu of current screening guidelines for diabetes, there continues to be a failure in accurate detection in over 50% of undiagnosed diabetes in Americans.[2]

Diabetes is a disease process characterized by a lack of effective insulin or no insulin production. Insulin is necessary to transport glucose out of the bloodstream to all of our cells. "Insulin is like a key that unlocks the doors of your cells so that glucose can get in and be used as a source of energy. Without insulin, extra glucose can't get into the cells and it stays in the blood."[4] Insulin is a hormone our body produces by beta cells in the pancreas. It is necessary to provide energy (glucose) for our bodies to function properly. The food we consume is broken down into glucose, also known as sugar, and is absorbed into the bloodstream. The serum glucose levels decrease when insulin moves sugar into the cells. The normal blood glucose range is between 70 and 180 mg/dL. When there are insufficient amounts of insulin, the serum glucose levels remain elevated thus enabling the development of diabetes.[5]

PREVALENCE/INCIDENCE

In 2050, it is estimated that 1 in 3 Americans will be diagnosed with diabetes, which will continue to overwhelm health care costs globally.[3] Inpatient hospitalizations are the main medical expenditures, not including medication costs. There is a "3 fold greater chance" for hospitalizations for people with diabetes.[3] Diabetes as a complicating factor accounts for the majority of inpatient admissions. Patients with diabetes are admitted with soft tissue and bone infections, strokes, urinary tract infections, renal failure, heart failure, and sepsis. Diabetes is a codriver for many admissions with attention to glycemic control.[6]

Diabetes is not as differentiated as other medical service lines. It is often captured in coding as a secondary diagnosis, with the infection or actual issue as the primary diagnosis. It is important to know that diabetes as an underlying comorbidity can increase acuity, costs, length of stay, and the risk of mortality. In order to accurately capture diabetes as a service line, hospitals should utilize coding to better account for direct health care costs and acuity of nursing care.

The coronavirus disease 2019 (COVID-19) pandemic has impacted the prevalence of diabetes more. Viral infections have been historically associated with the development of diabetes due to beta cell destruction leading to a lack of insulin production. Epidemiologic studies recognize the severity of COVID-19 and higher rates of new-onset diabetes and diabetic ketoacidosis after infection. Statistics vary; however, post-COVID-19 infection, the higher risk of developing new-onset diabetes has been between 11% and 276% and is dependent on age, severity of infection, timing of diagnoses, and different comparator groups.[7] The bidirectional relationship is known; however, it is too early to come to conclusions on the exact mechanism of how COVID-19 causes new-onset diabetes. More studies and research are needed to determine this. It is known that beta cells are tolerant to infection with severe SARS-CoV-2, which leads to their destruction. Unfortunately, beta cells do not regenerate resulting in impaired or no insulin production causing persistent hyperglycemia further developing into new-onset diabetes. The hyperglycemic effects of high-dose glucocorticoids for severe COVID-19 are also noted.[7]

NATURE OF THE PROBLEM

The International Hypoglycemia Study Group defined a leveling system for classification (**Table 1**). Level 1 is considered mild but requires further monitoring and ingestion of fast-acting carbohydrates if able to swallow. Level 2 is considered clinically

Table 1
Most recent professional societies' recommendations on Inpatient glycemic targets for older patients

Society, Year (Reference)	Critically III (mg/dL)	Noncritically III (mg/dL)		Notes Regarding Older Patients
		Fasting	Postprandial	
ADA/AACE,[9] 2009	110–180	100–140	100–180	No specific recommendations for older patients
International Diabetes Federation,[10] 2014	–	<140	<180	These targets are for older patients
Diabetes Canada,[11] 2018	110–180	90–140	<180	No specific recommendations for older patients
Endocrine Society,[23] 2019	–	100–140	140–180	These targets are for older patients
Joint British Diabetes, Societies for Inpatients Care,[24] 2019	140–180	140–180		100–216 mg/dL (6–12 mmol/L) is acceptable for older patients
American Diabetes Association,[12] 2020	140–180	140–180		No specific recommendations for older patients; >180 mg/dL (10.0 mmol/L) in patients with severe comorbidities

Data from Gosmanov AR, Mendez CE, Umpierrez GE. Challenges and Strategies for Inpatient Diabetes Management in Older Adults. *Diabetes Spectr.* 2020;33(3):227-235. https://doi.org/10.2337/ds20-0008.

significant as neurogenic symptoms and neuroglycopenia can occur. Confusion and mental status changes with disorientation are common. Treatment should be immediate with serial monitoring of blood glucose levels until recovered, usually until glucose is above 100 mg/dL. Level 3 is severe hypoglycemia. Emergent treatment includes intravenous dextrose and/or glucagon administration with continuous glucose infusions as needed. Aggressive care is indicated, including advanced life support measures if warranted[8] (see **Table 1**).

Hypoglycemia is the most common complication of hospitalized patients with diabetes.[8] Inpatient hypoglycemia is associated with negative clinical outcomes increasing the rate of mortality. Depending on the severity of the event, the patient could experience stroke, seizures, aspiration, respiratory failure requiring intubation with continuous mechanical ventilation, hypotension, and the need to transfer to a higher level of care. If the patient experiences severe hypoglycemia, the risk of mortality increases.[8] Significantly, "A 2.6% short-term mortality was found among hypoglycemic admissions."[8] Serial hypoglycemic events can increase the risk of strokes, acute coronary syndrome, and in-hospital falls. Increased length of stay can be attributed to hypoglycemia adding additional costs to the overall hospital stay. The Centers for Medicare and Medicaid, in 2019, classified severe hypoglycemia as a "never event," indicating severe hypoglycemia should never occur.[8]

The risk of mortality increases with hypoglycemia in patients with diabetes. Low blood glucose levels can cause cardiac arrhythmia leading to sudden cardiac death.[8,13] One study discovered that after a severe episode of hypoglycemia, the 3 year cumulative occurrence of coronary heart disease was 10.8%, and mortality was 28.3%.[8] Drug-induced hypoglycemia, if not promptly recognized and treated, leads to mortality.

Risk factors for inpatient hypoglycemia include the following: individual, management, and institutional factors. Individual factors consist of age, and comorbid conditions including impaired renal function, liver failure, malignancy, sepsis, anemia, heart failure, adrenal insufficiency, and thyroid disorders. Managing factors include hyperglycemia medications, variable dietary intake, and prolonged periods of nothing by mouth (NPO) status. Institutional factors include monitoring blood glucose, ambiguous medication dosing instructions, aggressive insulin therapy, discrepancies in dietary intake, the timing of meal trays with insulin administration, and inadequate coordination and communication between health care team members.[13]

Patients with impaired kidney function are prone to hypoglycemic excursions due, in part, to the severity of the injury. Patients with end-stage renal function are challenging to treat as insulin resistance occurs before dialysis and insulin degradation occurs postdialysis. Liver function abnormalities disrupt carbohydrate metabolism and glucogenesis.[13] Infections, especially sepsis and/or septic shock increase the risk of hypoglycemia.[13] Furthermore, oral medications can predispose patients to hypoglycemia, especially sulfonylureas. If renal function is impaired, the half-life of sulfonylureas is extended, causing refractory hypoglycemia.[14] Octreotide administered in subcutaneous injections, until glucose stabilizes, has been known to reverse the effects of sulfonylureas better than glucose alone. "Octreotide is a synthetic octapeptide analogue of somatostatin which can effectively suppress insulin secretion."[14] Recognizing sulfonylurea-induced hypoglycemia and starting octreotide promptly can improve patient outcomes and reduce mortality.[14] Additional oral medications inducing hypoglycemia include quinolone antibiotics, macrolide antibiotics, sulfa-based antibiotics, beta-blockers, angiotensin-converting enzyme inhibitors, and angiotensin receptor blockers. Obtaining a list of current home medications is critical for early interventions. Electronic pharmacy records are available for viewing in some electronic medical records systems.[8]

The following conditions increase the risk of hypoglycemia: Overbasalization of insulin, no reduction in home medication regimen, stacking effects of fast-acting pre-meal and scheduled correction with variable dietary intake, treatment of hyperkalemia in patients with end-stage renal disease, steroid tapering without adjusting insulin doses, full dose administration when the patient is in NPO status, and unknown sensitivity to insulin. Communication of point of care (POC) glucose results between nursing staff can lead to insulin administration delays, leading to hypoglycemia. Appreciating that glucose levels change hourly, it is important to ensure the administration of short-acting insulin within 30 minutes of the glucose result and long-acting insulin within 60 minutes to prevent subsequent hypoglycemia. Onset, peak, and duration are the primary drivers of balanced meal tray delivery, lack of nutritional intake, and other medications causing hyperglycemia.[8]

PATHOGENESIS

Diabetes mellitus is a metabolic disorder with complex pathogenesis differentiated by persistent hyperglycemia (**Fig. 1**). Insulin deficiencies, either resistance or lack of production, characterize diabetes. Insulin is produced in the beta cells of the pancreas and is responsible for allowing glucose to move from the bloodstream into the cells. When this does not happen and the blood glucose level remains elevated, greater than 180 mg/dL or higher, macrovascular and microvascular complications occur. The normal blood glucose levels are between 70 and 180 mg/dL. With inadequate insulin to regulate blood glucose levels, permanent end-organ damage occurs. Various body systems and organs include the autonomic and peripheral nervous systems, which include the eyes, the brain, the heart, the kidneys, the skin, and the feet. Chronic organ damage can result in renal failure, blindness, and severe neuropathy.[15]

TYPE 1 DIABETES MELLITUS

Type 1 diabetes is an autoimmune disorder that destroys the pancreatic beta cells, resulting in absolute insulin deficiency. The trigger for the immune system is not fully understood; however, environmental and genetic factors do play a role. Beta cell destruction is immune-mediated and has a sudden onset in infants and children.[15] For older adults, it can gradually increase to absolute insulin deficiency. It is not uncommon for a patient to be admitted with diabetic ketoacidosis (DKA) and discover they have diabetes. There are several autoantibodies associated with immune-mediated beta cell destruction. Glutamic acid decarboxylase autoantibodies include GAD65, islet cell autoantibodies (ICAs), including ICA512, tyrosine phosphates IA-2 and IA2a, insulin autoantibodies (IAAs), and lastly islet-specific zinc transporter isoform 8. GAD65 is the most definitive of the immune response.[15]

Laboratory results confirm the presence of the following autoantibodies at the time of diagnosis: GAD65 roughly 80%, then ICAs 69% to 90%, and IA-2a 54% to 75% of the time. It is notable that serum C-peptide levels are very low or nonexistent, indicating insulin deficiency. GAD65 is the most significant for diagnosing type 1 diabetes in adults. The IAAs are clinically significant for infants and young children who have not had insulin before presenting in about 70% of all infants and young children.[15]

Adults can develop type 1 diabetes, which is usually a slow progression of relative insulin deficiency until it becomes absolute abruptly. Adults with slow-progressing type 1 diabetes have been incorrectly diagnosed as having type 2 diabetes. The confirmatory diagnosis is made with the laboratory results revealing the presence of autoantibodies. New onset type 1 diabetes in adults is referred to as "latent autoimmune diabetes in adults (LADA)." LADA accounts for 2% to 12% of all diabetes in

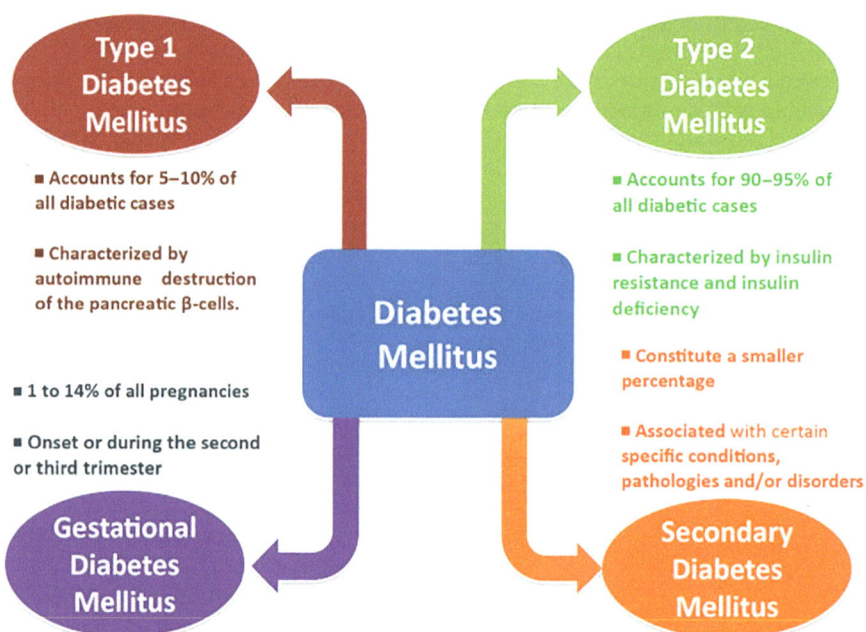

Fig. 1. Four types of diabetes mellitus. (*From* Banday MZ, Sameer AS, Nissar S. Pathophysiology of diabetes: An overview. Avicenna J Med. 2020;10(4):174-188. Published 2020 Oct 13. https://doi.org/10.4103/ajm.ajm_53_20).

adults.[15] Patients with LADA can often present as new onset type 2 diabetes. Intensive care unit (ICU) nurses should encourage follow-up with primary care physicians and endocrinologists postdischarge to ensure proper typing. In this post-COVID-19 world, testing for antibodies is becoming a must to ensure accurate typing for an accurate medication regimen. Type 2 medications prescribed to an adult with LADA have the potential to cause adverse effects. Outpatient antibody panels are not usually ordered as a part of inpatient hospitalization. Postdischarge follow-up is critical and should be a discussion point of inpatient diabetes education.

Patients with type 1 diabetes have more fluctuations in blood sugar making them more prone to sudden hypoglycemia. This is difficult to manage reactively. It is not uncommon to see hyperglycemia treated with insulin and then a subsequent drop in hypoglycemia levels.[15]

TYPE 2 DIABETES MELLITUS

Type 2 diabetes comprises 90% to 95% of all diabetes cases. It is characterized by insulin resistance and beta-cell dysregulation. Insulin resistance occurs when the peripheral cells no longer respond favorably to insulin and block glucose from leaving the bloodstream. There is an initial demand for beta cell hyperfunction, which leaves circulating insulin levels elevated. This is temporary and over time beta cell function decreases leading to insulin deficiency. Type 2 is a slow progression until the patient becomes symptomatic. It is important to note that annual A1C monitoring on an outpatient basis could catch new cases of type 2 before any diabetes symptoms appear. Polyuria, polydipsia, nocturia, unintentional weight loss, and visual changes are the most common symptoms. Type 2 is multifactorial including familial history, age, obesity, sedentary lifestyle, environmental factors, and other medical conditions including polycystic ovary syndrome. Gestational diabetes (GDM) is a predictive risk factor for the development of type 2 diabetes in later years.[16] A distinguishing characteristic is no immune system response. The presence of autoantibodies does not occur.[16] It is known more as a relative insulin deficiency as beta cell function gradually fades.

GESTATIONAL DIABETES

GDM occurs only in pregnancy, usually discovered in the second or third trimester by glucose screening tests. In the third trimester, blood glucose levels can rise to diabetes levels. Maternal insulin requirements increase as the "feto-placental unit" grows.[16] Maternal hormones increase insulin resistance. In 2014, the Centers for Disease Control and Prevention reported up to 9.2% of all pregnancies have GDM.[16] The goals of care for GDM are to remain normoglycemic during pregnancy and to prevent further development of diabetes in later years. Insulin is the preferred drug of treatment in the United States. Postdelivery maternal insulin requirements dramatically decrease once the placenta is delivered. Many mothers do not need any further insulin after delivery. GDM is primarily treated outpatient; however, inpatient care is necessary for complications including DKA, pre-eclampsia, infections, and dehydration.[16] Hypoglycemia can occur with GDM if the nutritional intake is poor and/or mismatched. Hypoglycemia in this population is defined as less than 60 mg/dL. After delivery, the traditional hypoglycemia of less than 70 mg/dL applies.

Pregnant patients with GDM can be admitted to an ICU for hypertension, pre-eclampsia with sequela, DKA, and other associated conditions. The ICU nurse should capture a detailed medical history, including the onset of diabetes, medication regimen, and names of maternal–fetal specialists and primary care physicians. Partnering with antepartum and/or labor and delivery nurses is essential to provide the best definitive care possible for the mother, which includes fetal outcomes.[15] Patients with existing diabetes before pregnancy can incur diabetes-related conditions during pregnancy including DKA. Care should be taken accordingly, and the ICU nurse should know this.

SECONDARY TYPES OF DIABETES MELLITUS

Maturity-onset diabetes of the young (MODY) is a genetically modified type most often noninsulin-dependent that originates with genetic modifications to specific genes involved in pancreatic beta cell function. The mutated genes on different chromosomes disrupt glucose sensing and insulin release. Most of these cases are diagnosed before 25 years of age, which often can be confused with type 1 diabetes. There is a strong familial history involving multiple generations with a traceable phenotype. Classifying which gene and chromosome comprises a number placed after the Y in MODY. MODY accounts for less than 2% of diabetes cases with the most common forms known as MODY2 and MODY3.[15] Inpatients with MODY are usually treated with insulin and can experience hypoglycemia.

Infections can cause beta cell dysfunction resulting in hyperglycemia, which develops into diabetes. As mentioned previously, it has been understood that certain viral infections can antagonize beta cell function. More drug-induced diabetes is becoming more common, unfortunately. Several different classes of medications are known to do this: glucocorticoids, thiazides, beta blockers, hormones relating to growth or thyroid function, protease inhibitors, and some antipsychotics.[15] It is possible to overcorrect unintentionally with the patient experiencing hypoglycemia.

INPATIENT HYPOGLYCEMIA

Inpatient guidelines for the treatment of hypoglycemia are usually initiated if blood glucose levels fall below 70 mg/dL. Hypoglycemia can occur before hospital arrival and be discovered on arrival at the emergency department. POC glucose testing is available for immediate testing upon arrival if suspected with subsequent treatment of intravenous dextrose solution for level 3 hypoglycemia. Level 1 and level 2 events may be treated with oral fruit juice.[13] Causal factors include taking antihyperglycemic medications without eating or delaying eating, failure of counterregulatory hormones, and severe infections including but not limited to sepsis and septic shock. Patients who respond quickly to treatment and can tolerate a meal are often discharged home with other appropriate therapies as needed. Patients with hypoglycemia are often admitted to a medical-surgical level of care if mild, and if persistent and refractory hypoglycemia, they are admitted to ICU.[13]

It is noted that 3% to 18% of hospitalized patients with diabetes have hypoglycemia, less than 70 mg/dL, with an increase in length of stay and risk of mortality. In this population, other adverse outcomes, such as falls and cardiovascular events, occur with increased frequency. Increased rates of seizures and coma for symptomatic hypoglycemia are noted.[13] Mild hypoglycemia can cause patients to experience fear, anxiety, and depression. Other medical conditions co-occurring include level of renal functioning, age, congestive heart failure, coronary artery disease, bacterial sepsis, respiratory failure, stroke, pancreatitis, intestinal issues, viral illnesses, and medication-induced.[13]

TREATMENT

Treatment with antihyperglycemic medications, including insulin, is a significant factor in determining hypoglycemic episodes. In insulin-naïve individuals, their sensitivity factor is not known. Not reducing home insulin dosages can also provoke unnecessary hypoglycemic events as nutritional intake is often lower than at home and frequent NPO status for procedures or surgeries. Weight-based insulin dosing is beneficial when compared to the current A1C level.[17] Patients aged 65 years and older with diabetes are more prone to hypoglycemia. They may need to have their home regimen reduced to 0.15 to 0.3 units/kg, body weight decreased further to 0.1 to 0.15 units/kg for those with renal failure defined as estimated glomerular filtrate rate less than 60, history of hypoglycemia or poor nutritional intake.[17] Treatment with insulin is the most common risk factor for hypoglycemia. Elderly adults are more susceptible to hypoglycemia due to failure of counterregulatory hormones, frailty, malnutrition, dementia, renal failure, and hypoglycemia unawareness.[18] Insulin therapy is preferred for managing hyperglycemia in the hospital regardless of age. For critically ill patients, intravenous infusion protocols are safe and effective, especially when treating DKA or hyperkinetic hyperosmolar syndrome (HHS). Postoperative cardiac bypass patients also receive intravenous insulin infusions. The Society of Critical Care Medicine recommends keeping blood glucose levels to 150 mg/dL or greater but less than 180 mg/dL to prevent hypoglycemia. Targets are outlined in **Table 2**.

PATIENT MONITORING AND SIDE EFFECTS

In the ICU, a variety of patients get admitted. Most of the time, patients are maintained NPO for a prolonged period (**Table 3**). Therefore, it is imperative to monitor blood glucose levels. Hypoglycemia has a higher incidence of occurrence in critical care

Table 2
Risk factors for inpatient hypoglycemia[9,12,19,20]

Patient factors	Advanced age
	Decreased renal function
	Low HbA1c
	High HbA1c in critically ill patients
	Long duration of diabetes
	Impaired hypoglycemia awareness
	Poor appetite/poor meal intake
	Chronic liver disease
Dosing and administration factors	Failure to adjust home diabetes regimen
	Aggressive diabetes management
	High basal dosing/basal only regimens
	Mismatch of POC BG testing with insulin dosing and meal delivery
	Inadequately addressed antecedent hypoglycemia
	Failure to account for dextrose-containing fluids
	Frequent insulin dosing and stacking of insulin action
	Failure to address changes in PO status
	Failure to address changes in steroid doses
	Use of nonstandard therapies: SU, premixed insulins, and concentrated insulins
	Use of correctional insulin overnight

Abbreviations: BG, blood glucose; HbA1c, hemoglobin A1c; PO, per os; POC, point of care; SU, sulfonylurea.

Data from Cruz P. Inpatient Hypoglycemia: The Challenge Remains. *Journal of Diabetes Science and Technology.* 2020;14(3):560-566. https://doi.org/10.1177/1932296820918540.

patients than in noncritical care patients because there is a higher level of acuity and multiple comorbidities, which makes them vulnerable to having consequences of electrolyte and hemodynamic changes.[19] Initially, doctors only want to frequently monitor the glucose levels of diabetics due to their sugar level fluctuations and being the highest risk for hypoglycemia,[20] but all ICU patients who are NPO should be monitored to prevent hypoglycemia. The frequency of glucose monitoring should depend on medication regimens, the type of diabetes a patient has, and even their overall health status. Glucose monitoring can be done at each meal and at the time of sleep, every 4 hours, every 2 hours, or even every hour, based on the patients' needs. In addition, when giving medications to correct hypoglycemia, glucose checks can be as frequent as every 20 minutes until the glucose level reaches an optimal value. The use of insulin and sulfonylurea regimens, fasting, or even food insecurity (patients' specialized diets, not liking hospital food, and so forth) can increase the risk of hypoglycemia.[9] Additionally, patients in the ICU are given an array of medications (steroids, norepinephrine, and dextrose drips) that can alter their glucose levels; doctors and pharmacists are

Table 3
International hypoglycemia classification

Level	Blood Glucose Range (mg/dL)	Clinical Characteristic
1	<70 but >54	Mild
2	<54	Significant
3	<40	Severe

proactive in treating hyperglycemia, but when these medications are discontinued, the insulin sliding scale should be adjusted. Alert patients should be educated on the drugs they are receiving and how they affect their glucose levels. Hypoglycemia can present itself with various symptoms like diaphoresis, confusion, trembling, dizziness, and even irritability; therefore, patients should be educated to alert medical staff of their symptoms so that their glucose levels can be checked. If patients are found to have low glucose levels, the nurses should act upon the results immediately to prevent further deterioration into a coma or death. Hypoglycemia can increase the risks of morbidity and mortality, increase the length of stays, and delay recovery.[19]

CHALLENGES WITH HYPOGLYCEMIA IN THE INTENSIVE CARE UNIT

Many challenges arise with critical care patients that affect hypoglycemia. Norepinephrine, or levophed, is a common medication used to treat low blood pressure, but a common side effect of the medication is peripheral vasoconstriction. This side effect can lead to discolored and cold fingers, ultimately altering the chemistry of the capillary blood used to collect a glucose sample. This blood sample could be altered, leading to pseudohypoglycemia; therefore, nurses would inaccurately treat the glucose level, which can lead to hyperglycemia.[21] Other etiologies affecting glucose readings are peripheral edema, peripheral vascular disease, hypoxemia, acidosis, hypotension, hematocrit levels, hypertriglyceridemia, and hyperbilirubinemia.[12] A challenge related to this is that nurses will run whole or arterial blood samples in a laboratory, but results can take a while to arrive, delaying care. However, some facilities do not have I-Stat analyzers to get results during POC or glucometers that are compatible with using blood aside from capillary blood. The nurse must also be able to communicate with other nurses and patient care technicians/certified nursing assistants on what the proper blood collection should be.

When patients are intubated and sedated, it can also be challenging for them to verbalize that they are having hypoglycemic symptoms; therefore, the nurses must use their critical thinking skills and assessment skills to recognize changes in patient's conditions to minimize critically low glucose levels (less than 40 mg/dL) (**Table 4**). Another challenge that arises with patients in critical care is the use of either hemodialysis or continuous renal replacement therapy. The kidneys are essential in clearing insulin and releasing glucose into the bloodstream; therefore, acute renal failure is associated with reduced kidney clearance, which can cause hypoglycemia.[21] Additionally, during hemodialysis, the exchange of fluids can decrease the plasma glucose concentration,[21] which can cause hypoglycemia; therefore, nurses should be proactive in checking glucose levels. Nurses should collaborate with physicians to adjust dialysate fluids that include sodium bicarbonate and glucose to reduce the prevalence of low glucose levels.

GOALS OF CARE (RECOVERY AFTER THE EVENT AND WHAT TO DO TO ELIMINATE AN EVENT BEFOREHAND)

Recognizing and treating hypoglycemia is imperative as it can lead to irreversible damage if not treated appropriately. To prevent a hypoglycemic event, there must be a multidisciplinary approach between critical care physicians, nurses, pharmacists, and even endocrinologists to identify and address underlying contributors to hypoglycemia.[20] In the ICU, patients can have many causes as to why hypoglycemia occurs like sepsis, organ failure, hepatic dysfunction, renal impairment, and wrongly dosed insulin therapy. Nurses should advocate for their patients and question medical regimens ordered for safety. It is important to prevent hypoglycemia because

Table 4 Blood glucose frequencies	
NPO	Every 4 h
Eating meals	qid before each meal and at bedtime
Tube feeding	Every 4 h
Total parenteral nutrition	Every 4 h
Intravenous insulin infusion	Every 1 h

Abbreviations: BG, blood glucose; NPO, nil per os; qid, 4 times a day.
   Data from Cruz P. Inpatient Hypoglycemia: The Challenge Remains. *Journal of Diabetes Science and Technology.* 2020;14(3):560-566. https://doi.org/10.1177/1932296820918540

frequent exposure to low blood sugar levels can increase the risk of stroke and has been associated with in-hospital falls.[8] Additionally, moderate guidelines state that hyperglycemia should not be treated intravenously unless glucose levels exceed 180 mg/dL.[19] Nurses and physicians should also be cognizant of ICU patients having stress-induced hyperglycemia due to acute illnesses; therefore, they should be aware that this spontaneously resolves when the stress of illness or inflammation resolves.[21] Furthermore, institutions should allow conscious and alert patients to manage their own insulin if they have insulin pumps to prevent hypoglycemic events.[21] In addition, continuous glucose monitoring systems (CGMs), not currently Food and Drug Administration (FDA)-approved for in-hospital use, did prove useful in the COVID-19 pandemic. CGMs have been used outpatient for trending glucose levels and detecting falls in glucose levels; therefore, they have been able to treat glucose levels proactively.[21] CGMG data are beneficial for trending glucose levels.

Critical care nurses must quickly resolve low blood sugar levels when patients have hypoglycemic events. Depending on the patient's status (alert or comatose), the nurse can give simple carbohydrates, glucagon (intramuscular or intravenous) or Dextrose 50% pushes to resolve the hypoglycemia and continue monitoring the glucose levels until the patient reaches a satisfactory range. If hypoglycemia persists, the root cause should be identified, but the patient will also need a solution that does not involve medication pushes or juices. Some doctors will order Dextrose 10% or Dextrose 5% Lactated Ringers to treat the hypoglycemia, and the nurse can titrate the Dextrose 10% solution until the patient reaches a normal glucose range. If patients are on insulin and suffer a hypoglycemic event, the insulin regimens should be evaluated and adjusted to prevent hypoglycemic events from occurring again.[19] Oral antihyperglycemic agents are not recommended in the inpatient setting, but patients will be on these medications before their ICU admission.[19] It is noted that some oral medications may be restarted after a downgrade from the ICU level of care, especially if the patient was on them before admission and the medication is in the hospital formulary. Therefore, it is important to review medication histories for all different classes of oral diabetes medications. If patients are found to be taking sulfonylureas, this can cause hypoglycemia because of their prolonged half-life, and octreotide should be used to suppress insulin secretions.[14]

SUMMARY

Patients with diabetes represent 38% of the patient population in community hospitals throughout the United States.[11] Hypoglycemia is defined as less than 70 mg/dL. Patients with hypoglycemia are at more risk for clinically adverse outcomes including death. Critical care nurses must recognize the signs and symptoms of hypoglycemia and initiate prompt intervention to reduce the risk of mortality.[10] Differentiating the types of diabetes is essential to advocate for accurate treatment regimens while hospitalized. Critical care nurses should be familiar with the following: type 1, type 1 LADA, type 2, GDM, MODY, and other causes of diabetes. Unless the patient is admitted for DKA or HHS, the primary reason for admission is likely not for glycemic control; however, in patients with all types of diabetes, glycemic control is always a primary driver of care. Future considerations for in-hospital management include using CGM as soon as the FDA approves. Identifying glucose trends and treating them proactively can reduce the length of stay and adverse events, including hypoglycemia, and lower mortality risk.

CLINICS CARE POINTS

- Diabetes is a worldwide health crisis.
- In 2024, it is predicted that 1.4 million people will be diagnosed.
- By 2050, it is predicted that 1 in 3 will be diagnosed.
- Diabetes is an insulin deficiency.
- Mortality risk is increased in people with diabetes.
- Hospitalized patients with diabetes can experience hypoglycemia suddenly.
- Standard of care dictates the quick, prompt treatment of hypoglycemia.
- Critically ill patients in the hospital can pose challenges in treating hypoglycemia.
- Severe hypoglycemia can cause permanent harm including mortality.
- The goal of care should be to prevent hypoglycemia when possible.

DISCLOSURE

The authors have nothing to disclose.

REFERENCES

1. American Diabetes Association. Newly diagnosed with diabetes. 2024. Available at: https://diabetes.org/living-with-diabetes/newly-diagnosed.
2. Rowley WR, Bezold C, Ectera AY. Diabetes 2030: insights from yesterday, today, and future trends. Popul Health Manag 2017;20(1):6–12.
3. Dhatariya K, Corsino L, Unpierrez G. Management of diabetes and hyperglycemia in hospitalized patients. In: Feingold KR, Anawalt B, Blackman RN, et al, editors. Endotext [Internet]. South Dartmouth (MA): MDText.com, IOnc; 2020. p. 200. Available at: https://www.ncbi.nlm.nih.gov/books/NBK279093/.
4. NovoCare. What is Diabetes?. Available at: factsheet_What_Is_Diabetes.pdf (novocare.com).
5. NovoCare. Understanding diabetes. 2024. Available at: Understanding Diabetes | NovoCare® Diabetes Education.
6. Hanover L. What are the most common reasons for hospital admissions for patients with diabetes? AJMC 2021. Available at: https://www.ajmc.com/view/what-are-the-most-common-reasons-for-hospital-admissions-for-patients-with-diabetes.

7. Perakakis N, Harb H, Hale BG, et al. Mechanisms and clinical relevance of the bidirectional relationship of viral infections with metabolic diseases. Lancet Diabetes Endocrinol 2023;11(6). Available at: https://www.clinicalkey.com/#!/content/journal/1-s2.0-S2213858723001547.

8. Cruz P. Inpatient hypoglycemia: the challenge remains. J Diabetes Sci Technol 2020;14(3):560–6.

9. Silbert R, Salcido-Montenegro A, Rodriguez-Gutierrez R, et al. Hypoglycemia among patients with type 2 diabetes: epidemiology, risk factors, and prevention Strategies. Curr Diab Rep 2018;18:53.

10. Mathew P, Thoppil D. Hypoglycemia. 2022. In: StatPearls [Internet]. Treasure Island (FL): StatPearls Publishing; 2024.

11. Seley JJ. Diabetes care in the inpatient setting. In: Childs BP, Cypress M, Spoliett GR, editors. Complete nurse's guide to diabetes care. 3rd edition. Arlington VA: American Diabetes Association; 2017.

12. Sreedharan R, Martini A, Das G, et al. Clinical challenges of glycemic control in the intensive care unit: a narrative review. World J Clin Cases 2022;10(31):11260–72.

13. Pratiwi C, Mokoagow MI, Made Kshanti IA, et al. The risk factors of inpatient hypoglycemia: a systematic review. Heliyon 2020;6(5):e03913.

14. Zafar S, Mahali LP, Ahsan H. Role of octreotide in sulfonylurea-induced hypoglycemia. J Endocr Soc 2021;5(Suppl 1):A396–7.

15. Banday MZ, Sameer AS, Nissar S. Pathophysiology of diabetes: an overview. Avicenna J Med 2020;10(4):174–88.

16. Homko CJ. Women and diabetes. In: Complete nurse's guide to diabetes care. 3rd edition. VA: American Diabetes Association Arlington; 2017. p. 436–44.

17. Khan S, Golden SH, Mathioudakis N. Associations between home insulin dose adjustments and glycemic outcomes at hospital admission. Diabetes Res Clin Pract 2017;127:51–8.

18. Gosmanov AR, Mendez CE, Umpierrez GE. Challenges and Strategies for inpatient diabetes management in older adults. Diabetes Spectr 2020;33(3):227–35.

19. Robinson A, Mathiason MA, Manchester C, et al. Evaluation of nurse-driven management of hypoglycemia in critically ill patients. Am J Crit Care 2024;33(3):218–25.

20. Mathew P, Thoppil D, McClinton T. Hypoglycemia (nursing). 2022. Available at: https://www.ncbi.nlm.nih.gov/books/NBK568695/.

21. Crespo JCL, Gomes VR, Barbosa RL, et al. Haemodialysis, nutritional disorders and hypoglycaemia in critical care. Br J Nurs 2017;26(5):281–6.

Current Recommendations for Insulin Therapy in the Hospitalized Patient

Charmaine D. Rochester-Eyeguokan, PharmD, BCACP, CDCES[a],*,
Kathleen J. Pincus, PharmD, BCPS, BCACP, CDCES[b]

KEYWORDS

- Insulin • Hospitalized patients • Nursing • Critical care

KEY POINTS

- Use insulin protocols with basal, mealtime, and correction insulin dosing in the hospitalized patient.
- For preoperative surgery, aim for hemoglobin A1c less than or equal to 8% and blood glucose less than or equal to 180 mg/dL for better postoperative outcomes.
- Effectively manage diabetes medications during transitions of care.

BACKGROUND

Stress-induced hyperglycemia is common in hospitalized and critically ill patients, with or without diabetes mellitus (DM). Up to 25% of hospitalized patients without DM experience hyperglycemia.[1] Over 30% of non-critically ill-hospitalized patients have DM.[1] Dysglycemia, including hypoglycemia, hyperglycemia, and blood glucose variability (GV), increases morbidity and mortality in all patients and must be prevented with evidence-based patient care.[2] In 2021, 1 DM-related death occurred every 5 seconds worldwide.[3] Of note, Medicare does not pay for hospital-acquired diabetic ketoacidosis (DKA), hyperglycemic hyperosmolar non-ketotic syndrome (HHNS), or hypoglycemia coma as these are preventable with implementation of evidence-based guidelines.[4]

Insulin is the best way to control persistent hyperglycemia greater than or equal to 180 mg/dL in hospitalized patients.[5–7] Before insulin initiation, consider the patient's

[a] Department of Practice, Sciences, and Health Outcomes Research (PSHOR), University of Maryland School of Pharmacy, 110 North Pine Street, Room 105E, Baltimore, MD 21201, USA;
[b] Department of Practice, Sciences, and Health Outcomes Research, University of Maryland School of Pharmacy, 20 North Pine Street, Room N425, Baltimore, MD 21201, USA
* Corresponding author. Department of Practice, Sciences, and Health Outcomes Research, University of Maryland School of Pharmacy, 110 North Pine Street, Room 105E, Baltimore, MD 21201.
E-mail address: crochest@rx.umaryland.edu

Crit Care Nurs Clin N Am 37 (2025) 117–131
https://doi.org/10.1016/j.cnc.2024.05.004
0899-5885/25/Published by Elsevier Inc.

type and duration of DM, prior insulin and non-insulin therapies, insulin resistance, HbA1c levels, blood glucose (BG) levels, and oral intake.[5] This article guides nurses in managing insulin in hospitalized patients. The use of insulin drips in the management of newly diagnosed patients with Type 1 diabetes mellitus (T1DM), DKA, and HHNS is discussed elsewhere.

GLYCEMIC GOALS

The NICE-SUGAR trial found that critically ill patients managed intensively (BG target 80–110 mg/dL) had no significant treatment advantage but a slightly higher risk of mortality and hypoglycemia, compared with those with a moderate glycemic goal (140–180 mg/dL).[8] Therefore, glycemic targets in hospitals are more relaxed than in outpatient settings. Expert guidelines recommend glycemic goals for critically and non-critically ill patients as follows:[5–7]

- BG greater than 180 mg/dL should prompt active insulin management.
- Elective surgery within 4 hours: goal A1c less than 8% and BG 100 to 180 mg/dL
- Critically ill patients: goal BG 140 to 180 mg/dL (American Diabetes Association) or 140 to 200 mg/dL (Society of Critical Care Medicine)
- Non-critically ill patients: goal BG 100 to 180 mg/dL
- Terminally ill patients and those with advanced kidney disease: BG up to 250 mg/dL.[5–7]

INSULIN OVERVIEW

Insulin products vary in source, onset, duration, concentration, and delivery method. Hospitals limit formulary options to mitigate medication errors. Understanding product differences is essential for patients transitioning from preadmission regimens (**Table 1**).

INSULIN PRODUCTS AND PHARMACOKINETICS

Human insulins are produced using *Escherichia coli* bacteria and mimic natural insulin, while insulin analogs are modified using recombinant deoxyribinucleic acid technology.[10,11] Human insulins are less expensive, but insulin analogs have more favorable glucose-lowering properties.[10,11]

Insulin products are categorized as ultra-rapid, rapid, short, intermediate, long, and ultra-long acting based on their onset and duration of action. Ultra-rapid, rapid, and short-acting insulins are used for mealtime coverage and correction doses and should be administered within 15 to 30 minutes of a meal. Equivalent dosing can be used when transitioning between ultra-rapid and rapid-acting insulin products, but certain products have prolonged duration of response. When transitioning between ultra-rapid or rapid insulin and short-acting insulin, adjust the timing of administration, and monitor changes in glycemic control during the 4 to 12 hours post-dose period. Exercise caution and closely monitor the patient's response to ensure optimal glycemic control is achieved.

Basal insulin can be intermediate, long, and ultra-long-acting. Insulin Neutral Protamine Hagedorn (NPH) is an intermediate-acting insulin with a duration of action of approximately 13 hours.[11,12] Basal insulin analogs have duration of action of greater than 24 hours, allow for once-daily dosing, and have no or minimal peaks to avoid mid-day hypoglycemia. Insulin Degludec is the only Food and Drug Administration-approved ultra-long-acting insulin with a duration of 42 hours, administered once daily for less GV and more flexibility in dosing timing.[11–13] Most basal insulin analogs can be interchanged on a unit-for-unit basis.

Table 1
Insulin types and pharmacokinetics[9]

Generic Name	Brand Name(s)	Concentration	Onset of Action	Peak Activity	Duration of Effect	Injection Schedule
Ultra-Rapid Acting						
Insulin Aspart	Fiasp	U-100	15 min	1 h	5–7 h	Start of meal
Insulin Lispro aabc	Lyumjev	U-100	15 min	1 h	4.6–7.3 h	Start of meal
Insulin Human	Afreeza	U-100	15 min	1 h	2.5–3 h	Inhaled; start of meal
Rapid Acting						
Insulin Glulisine	Apidra	U-100	15 min	1 h	3–4 h	Within 15 min of meals
Insulin Aspart	Novolog	U-100	15 min	1 h	3–5 h	Within 5–10 min of meals
Insulin Lispro	Humalog	U-100 U-200	15 min	1 h	5.7–6.7 h	Within 15 min of meal
	Admelog	U-100	15 min	1 h	6–9 h	Within 15 min of meal
Short Acting						
Insulin Regular	Novolin R	U-100	30 min	2–3 h	4–12 h	Within 30 min of meal
	Humulin R	U-100	30 min	2–3 h	4–12 h	Within 30 min of meal
	Humulin R	U-500	30 min	2–3 h	13–24 h	Within 30 min of meal
Intermediate Acting						
Insulin Neutral Protamine Hagedorn (NPH)	Novolin N	U-100	1–2 h	4–6 h	14–24 h	Usually at bedtime or twice daily with regular insulin
	Humulin N	U-100	1–2 h	4–6 h	14–24 h	Usually at bedtime or twice daily with regular insulin
Long Acting						
Insulin Glargine	Lantus	U-100	1–3 h	No Peak	>24 h	Once daily (same time each day)
	Basaglar	U-100	1–3 h	No peak	24 h	Once daily (same time each day)
	Toujeo	U-300	6 h	No peak	36 h	Once daily (same time each day)
Insulin Glargine yfgn	Semglee	U-100	1–3 h	No peak	>24 h	Once daily (same time each day)
	Rezvoglar	U-100	1–3 h	No peak	>24 h	Once daily (same time each day)

(continued on next page)

Table 1
(continued)

Generic Name	Brand Name(s)	Concentration	Onset of Action	Peak Activity	Duration of Effect	Injection Schedule
Insulin Detemir[a]	Levemir	U-100	1 h	3–14 h	6–23 h	Once daily or every 12 h
Ultra-Long Acting						
Insulin Degludec	Tresiba	U-100 U-200	1 h	No peak	42 h	Once daily
Mixed Insulins						
Insulin Aspart Protamine & Insulin Aspart	Novolog Mix 70/30	U-100	60–90 min	4–12 h	18–24 h	2 divided doses within 15 min of meals
Insulin Lispro Protamine & Insulin Lispro	Humalog Mix 75/25 Humalog Mix 50/50	U-100	60–90 min	4–12 h	18–24 h	2 divided doses within 15 min of meals
NPH & Regular Insulin	Novolin 70/30 Humulin 70/30	U-100	60–90 min	4–12 h	14–24 h	2 divided doses within 30–45 min of meals

[a] Insulin (detemir) will phase out of the US market in December 2024.
Adapted from PharMerica corporation. Insulin – Comparison Chart. https://pharmerica.com/wp-content/uploads/2022/05/DidYouKnow_Insulin_Insulin-Comparison-Chart_04.2022.pdf. Accessed 15 Feb 2024.

Pre-mixed insulin products combine rapid or short-acting and intermediate-acting insulin, limiting dose titration, and increasing the risk of hypoglycemia. They are not recommended for in-hospital use. Combination products of long-acting insulin with once-daily Glucagon-Like Peptide-1 Receptor Agonists (GLP1 RAs) are available including Insulin Glargine/Lixisenatide (Soliqua) and Insulin Degludec/Liraglutide (Xultophy).[9]

Concentrated insulin products like Insulin Lispro U-200, Insulin Degludec U-200, Insulin Glargine U-300, and Insulin Regular U-500 reduce injection volume but are considered high-risk medications with the potential for serious hypoglycemia with dosing errors.[14] They are available in a Kwik Pen device demarcated by units to limit dosing errors. Human Regular U-500 insulin is also available in 20-mL multidose vials, which must be prescribed and dispensed with specific U-500 syringes that are demarcated by units to avoid confusion. Careful confirmation of home doses is necessary as patients may quote units and milliliters interchangeably.

When switching to or from Insulin Glargine U-300, dose titration is necessary. Consider a 20% dose reduction when transitioning from Insulin Glargine U-300 to a U-100 analog, or from the total daily dose (TDD) of a twice-daily NPH to basal insulin analog. When transitioning from basal insulin to insulin NPH, a unit-for-unit conversion is reasonable based on glycemic control and hypoglycemia risk.[15]

INSULIN ADMINISTRATION

Insulin administration occurs through subcutaneous, intravenous, inhalation, or pump methods. Avoid administering insulin intramuscularly due to potentially severe hypoglycemia.[16] Insulin for injection comes in vials and pre-filled pens. Vials are less expensive but require more steps. Pre-filled pens are easier to use but require specific needles. Proper education is needed for both methods. Intravenous insulin infusions are used in critical care, perioperative settings, and for the treatment of DKA. They are managed through protocols with predefined infusion rates and use rapid or short-acting insulins.

An insulin inhalation device called Afrezza delivers ultra-rapid-acting insulin for mealtime use but causes local irritation and is contraindicated in patients with chronic lung disease and lung cancer.[17]

Insulin can be administered through pumps, continuous subcutaneous insulin infusions (CSII), sensor-augmented pumps, or automated insulin delivery (AID) systems. Insulin pumps deliver rapid-acting insulin through a cannula to cover basal and bolus needs.[18] CSII are disposable patch-like devices that deliver rapid-acting insulin continuously throughout the day to cover basal insulin needs. Some of these devices can also deliver bolus insulin to cover mealtime requirements.[18] Augmented insulin pumps use continuous glucose monitoring (CGM) to temporarily stop the insulin infusion when glucose is low or predicted to go low. AID systems can also adjust basal insulin rates or provide correction doses based on CGM.[18] Insulin pumps and AID systems are recommended for patients with T1DM, as well as patients with Type 2 Diabetes (T2DM) who require multiple daily insulin injections.

INITIATING INSULIN DOSAGES IN NON-CRITICALLY ILL-HOSPITALIZED PATIENTS

For optimal outcomes, non-critically ill-hospitalized patients with poor intake or those taking nothing by mouth should receive basal insulin or a basal plus bolus insulin plan. However, most non-critically ill-hospitalized patients with adequate nutritional intake should have an insulin plan containing basal, prandial, and correction components to their plan.[5]

Basal Doses

Basal insulin is administered to patients during fasting to control gluconeogenesis once daily in the morning or at bedtime for insulin glargine or insulin degludec. Insulin Detemir can be given once or twice daily but this insulin will phase out of the United States market in December 2024. NPH can be given twice daily or at bedtime.[19]

Bolus or Prandial Doses

Bolus insulin is appropriate to cover carbohydrate intake and is used with dextrose in IV fluids, tube feeds, and total parenteral nutrition (TPN). For patients using insulin pumps or CSII, bolus administration is utilized around mealtime.

Correctional Doses

Correctional dosing is provided to decrease hyperglycemia to the target range usually below 150 mg/dL premeal, or 200 mg/dL at bedtime. Appropriate insulin includes ultra-rapid-acting, rapid-acting, or short-acting insulin.[19] A correctional dose is different from a sliding scale because it is a small incremental insulin increase to correct premeal hyperglycemia compared to a traditional sliding scale insulin, which is not beneficial and is associated with dysglycemia.[20,21] Some authors have published samples of correctional dose scales elsewhere.[20,22,23]

Correction dosing protocols are based on anticipated insulin sensitivity, with higher doses often needed in patients with T2DM, increased body weight, and higher TDD insulin. In the hospital, correction doses are often timed with pre-meal BG readings and bolus insulin administration. The dose administered to the patient is an additive of the correction dose, to correct for pre-meal hyperglycemia, and the scheduled mealtime dose, to cover the anticipated glucose load. If a patient needs frequent correction doses, their current basal insulin dose may not be sufficient, or their mealtime insulin did not adequately cover the previous meal. Consider reviewing their insulin dosing for potential adjustments. The use of correction dosing alone is not recommended.[5]

TYPE 2 DIABETES

Basal doses should provide consistent coverage throughout the day and are best assessed through fasting BG levels. Initiating insulin in non-critically ill patients with T2DM involves calculating a TDD, dividing it between basal and bolus doses, and documenting a correction dose regimen. The TDD can be calculated using 1 of 4 methods: home-based regimen, correction doses, insulin drip, and weight-based regimen.[22] For the home-based regimen, the TDD includes basal and bolus insulin doses used in 24 hours. The full TDD is used for patients who are hyperglycemic on admission or those with physiologic stressors like infections, while 75% of the TDD is used for elderly and hypoglycemic patients.[22] Clinicians can sum the units a patient on correction dose-only regimen used in the last 24 hours to calculate the TDD. For patients on an insulin drip, the clinician can multiply the total units used in the last 4 hours by 6 to give the TDD.

The weight-based regimen varies based on insulin sensitivity ranging from 0.25 to 3 units/kg/day for patients with low insulin sensitivity ($\leq$40 units), 0.4 units/kg/day for patients with moderate insulin sensitivity (40–80 units daily), and 0.5 to 1 unit/kg/day for patients with insulin resistance (>80 units daily).[20,22,24] Patients with low insulin sensitivity are lean, malnourished, take nothing by mouth, have a poor appetite, a history of hypoglycemia, elderly greater than 70 years, insulin naïve, and have chronic kidney disease (estimated glomerular filtration rate [eGFR] <45 mL/min/1.73 m^2) or are on dialysis. Patients with moderate insulin sensitivity are usually T1DM patients who are not recently diagnosed. Patients with insulin resistance include patients with obesity (Body mass index [BMI] >35 kg/m^2), on corticosteroids, or have postoperative stress or infections.[22]

To optimize results, one can distribute the TDD dose as 50% basal insulin and 50% bolus or prandial insulin then divide rapid-acting insulin into 3 equal doses before each meal. The insulin should be adjusted based on bedside BG measurements.[22]

TYPE 1 DIABETES

Estimate the TDD in patients with T1DM based on weight (0.4–1 unit/kg/day) with higher doses required during the diagnosis of DKA or T1DM patients, puberty, menses, and medical illness, and use lower doses (0.2–0.6 units/kg) in young children and those in the honeymoon period. Typically, 0.5 units/kg/day is used with approximately one-half of the TDD as basal and the other as prandial insulin.[25] Patients with T1DM must always have basal, bolus, and correction dosing as part of their regimen. To minimize hypoglycemia, use insulin analogs, consider a CSII and a continuous glucose monitor (CGM) at the time of diagnosis, and educate patients on correction doses and matching mealtime insulin doses to carbohydrate intake.[25]

NON-INSULIN TREATMENTS

There are multiple non-insulin treatments used for patients with T2DM (**Table 2**).[5,18,26] Many of these will be held on hospital admission, but nurses can monitor for adverse drug effects and advocate for the appropriate inclusion of these agents in discharge treatment plans. Metformin, a biguanide, is well-tolerated but can lead to gastrointestinal side effects including nausea, diarrhea, and stomach cramping, especially during dose titration. It can also increase the risk of lactic acidosis, though incidence remains rare. To reduce this risk, metformin is contraindicated in patients with eGFR less than 30 mL/min/m^2, and caution is recommended in patients with eGFR 30 to 45 mL/min/ m^2. As acute kidney injury is more likely, metformin is often discontinued on hospital admission. If renal and volume status is adequate, it can be restarted on discharge.

Sodium-glucose cotransporter 2 inhibitors (SGLT2i) increase the urinary elimination of glucose. Due to this mechanism, SGLT2i use is associated with increased risks of urinary tract and genital mycotic infections. Due to the large molecular size of glucose, SGLT2i also has a diuretic effect, which can lead to decreased volume status and blood pressure. SGLT2i has shown improved renal outcomes in patients with chronic and diabetic kidney disease and reduced rates of major atherosclerotic cardiovascular events (MACE) in patients with high atherosclerotic cardiovascular disease (ASCVD) risk. SGLT2i are recommended to be held 3 to 4 days before planned surgeries. All available SGLT2i have shown improved outcomes in patients with heart failure (HF); therefore, clinicians can continue SGLT2i during hospitalization for patients with HF.

GLP1 is an incretin mimetic hormone released in response to meals that trigger the release of preformed insulin, slows gastric emptying time, and improves satiety. Dipeptidyl peptidase 4 (DPP4) is the enzyme that degrades naturally produced GLP1. Available antihyperglycemic options targeting this system include synthetic GLP1 RAs, DPP4 inhibitors, and GLP1 RA combined with glucose-dependent insulinotropic polypeptide (GIP). GIP is another incretin hormone that increases insulin and glucagon release while decreasing hunger. GLP1 RAs have demonstrated weight reduction, slowed progression of kidney disease, and reduced MACE rates in patients at high ASCVD risk. The dual GLP1 RA/GIP product has shown significant weight reduction, with studies on other patient-oriented outcomes ongoing. DPP4 inhibitors

Table 2
Non-insulin treatment options[5,18,26]

Therapeutic Class	Products	Mechanism of Action	Benefits	Side Effects	Renal Dose Adjustments Needed	Perioperative Recommendations
Biguanides	Metformin	Block gluconeogenesis Enhance insulin sensitivity	High efficacy Low cost	Gastrointestinal Vitamin B12 deficiency	Yes	Hold day of surgery
Sodium-Glucose Cotransporter 2 (SGLT2) Inhibitors	Canagliflozin Dapagliflozin Empagliflozin Ertugliflozin	Reduce renal glucose reabsorption	Intermediate-high efficacy Intermediate weight loss Cardiovascular benefit[a] Renal benefit[b]	Urinary tract infections Genital mycotic infections Diabetic ketoacidosis Dehydration Hypotension	Yes	Hold 3–4 days before surgery; restart when food intake is resumed
Glucagon-like Peptide 1 Receptor Agonists (GLP1 RAs)	Dulaglutide Exenatide Liraglutide Semaglutide	Delay gastric emptying time Increase sensation of satiety Increase insulin release	High-very high efficacy Intermediate-very high weight loss Cardiovascular benefit[a] Renal benefit[b]	Gastrointestinal Ileus Pancreatitis Gallbladder disease Thyroid cancer	No	Hold 1 dose (either daily or weekly) before surgery[27]
Dual Glucose-Dependent Insulinotropic Polypeptide (GIP) and GLP1 RAs	Tirzepatide	Delay gastric emptying time Increase sensation of satiety Increase insulin release	Very high efficacy Very high weight loss	Gastrointestinal Ileus Pancreatitis Gallbladder disease Thyroid cancer Gastroparesis	Yes	Hold 1 dose (weekly) before surgery[27]
Dipeptidyl Peptidase 4 (DPP-4) Inhibitors	Alogliptin Linagliptin Saxagliptin Sitagliptin	Block breakdown of endogenous GLP-1	Intermediate efficacy	Pancreatitis Joint pain	Yes	Do not hold
Thiazolidinediones (TZDs)	Pioglitazone	Enhance insulin sensitivity	High efficacy Low Cost	Weight gain Increased heart failure risks Fluid retention	No	Do not hold
Sulfonylureas	Glimepiride Glipizide Glyburide	Increase insulin secretion	High efficacy Low cost	Risk of hypoglycemia Weight gain	Caution	Hold day of surgery

[a] Cardiovascular benefit–reduction of major atherosclerotic cardiovascular events (MACE) or improved heart failure outcomes have been demonstrated for specific agents within this class.
[b] Reduction in progression of kidney disease has been demonstrated for specific agents within this class.

have shown no excess cardiovascular risk, except an increased risk of hospitalizations with saxagliptin. The American Society of Anesthesiologists released a consensus statement recommending GLP1 RAs be held for 1 dose; either 1 day for daily medications or 1 week for weekly medications, before surgery.[27] DPP4 inhibitors need not be held before surgeries, regardless of fasting.

Thiazolidinediones (TZDs) increase insulin sensitivity in peripheral muscle and fat cells. The most significant side effect is fluid retention, which can lead to weight gain, edema, or HF exacerbations. TZDs are contraindicated in patients with HF for this reason.

Sulfonylureas (SU) act on the pancreatic beta-cells to increase insulin production. As this mechanism is not glucose-dependent, SU confers the highest risk of hypoglycemia of the non-insulin treatment options. Glyburide has active metabolites which are also renally cleared, leading to increased risk of hypoglycemia in patients with impaired renal function. Perioperative recommendations usually involve holding the day of surgery when fasting is indicated. It is recommended to discontinue all other oral antihyperglycemic medications (eg, alpha-glucosidase inhibitors, meglitinides, and bromcriptine) on hospital admission.

SPECIAL CLINICAL CONSIDERATIONS
Pre-operative Insulin Adjustment

Prior to surgery, insulin doses are often decreased to reduce the risk of hypoglycemia during pre-operative fasting. Reductions of 20% to 25% for basal insulin analogs or 50% for insulin NPH the morning of the surgery are recommended.[28] Larger basal dose reductions of 50% to 75% can be considered for patients with a high-risk of hypoglycemia or insulin resistance.[28] While fasting, basal insulin should be continued and prandial insulin doses held with monitoring and administration of correction doses every 4 to 6 hours.[5,28]

Post-Operative Considerations

Patients may experience elevated BG after surgery due to increased insulin resistance and endogenous glucose production as part of the body's stress response.[26] Hyperglycemia can also lead to poor surgical outcomes through impaired wound healing and immune response.[26] As such, insulin requirements may vary post-operatively. Frequent BG monitoring with correction doses is advised. Mealtime insulin doses should be restarted as the patient resumes normal oral intake.

Specialized Nutrition and Insulin

Hyperglycemia is common in patients receiving TPN due to pre-existing DM, hyperglycemia, dextrose infusion rates, critical illness, and acute stress responses.[29,30] Hyperglycemia is also common in up to one-third of patients with enteral nutrition (EN).[31]

Regular human insulin is the only recommended insulin for the addition to TPN due to its stability and ability to control hyperglycemia during TPN.[32] Adjust insulin dose according to changes in dextrose to prevent dysglycemia. The daily insulin dosage for the TPN may be determined at a rate of 1 unit per 10 to 15 g of dextrose and included in the TPN. If glycemic goals are not met, adjust the dosage by 0.5 units per 10 g of dextrose daily.[5,33]

Regarding EN, it is recommended to administer rapid- or short-acting insulin subcutaneously at a rate of 1 unit per 10 to 15 g of carbohydrate, before the initiation of daily feedings. NPH insulin can be administered along with feeding patients on nocturnal tube feedings to cover the glucose load.[5] If EN therapy is discontinued, initiate an intravenous glucose infusion immediately, to prevent hypoglycemia. To maintain glycemic control in patients on EN, it is recommended that regular monitoring be conducted, and correctional doses of insulin administered, as necessary.[5]

Glucocorticoid Therapy and Insulin

Corticosteroids cause hyperglycemia in most patients, whether they have DM or not.[5] When intermediate-acting steroids like prednisone, prednisolone, methylprednisolone, or triamcinolone are given once daily in the morning, the peak BG level can be alleviated by a single dose of NPH insulin. If an intermediate-acting steroid is given twice daily, NPH should be given concomitantly.[22] For patients already on a basal-bolus regimen, some clinicians recommend adding NPH as a third insulin to adjust for steroid tapers. In this way, both the steroid and NPH will be discontinued simultaneously, and the patient will remain with the stable basal-bolus regimen. Initiate 5 units of NPH in patients without diabetes while patients with diabetes can use 10 units. If the patient is not on basal-bolus insulin, NPH with correction insulin should be used. NPH insulin should be held once the prednisone is held.[22]

For individuals taking long-acting glucocorticoids, undergoing high-dose dexamethasone therapy, or utilizing multidose or continuous glucocorticoids, managing basal and premeal readings will require high doses of long-acting basal-bolus regimens, correction insulin, or even an insulin drip for uncontrolled hyperglycemia. Consistent monitoring is essential.[5,22]

INSULIN SELF-MANAGEMENT: INSULIN PUMPS AND CONTINUOUS GLUCOSE MONITORING

Individuals who are acutely ill, but cognitively and physically stable, and want to continue performing self-care in the hospital should do so. On the other hand, some clinicians express concerns for inpatient use of CGM including the accuracy of CGM data during acute physiologic disturbances (eg, hypoxemia, vasoconstriction, severe dehydration, and rapidly changing glucose concentrations in DKA), as well as chemical interference with BG readings (eg, high doses of acetaminophen [>4 g], salicylic acid, and ascorbic acid).[34] The Joint Commission has published guidance on the development of policies and procedures to guide safe usage of these devices inpatient.[35] These include considerations for changes in patient condition, availability of replacement medication and batteries, and device damage or failure.[35] These policies may include nurse supervision of medication and device storage, confirmatory testing with hospital calibrated glucose meters, and documentation of patient self-testing results in the medical record. Care must be taken to identify insulin pump errors including cannula dislodgement and tube occlusion promptly, as these can lead to abrupt cessation of insulin delivery and adverse patient outcomes.

TRANSITIONS OF CARE & SYSTEM-BASED INTERVENTIONS

Given the high-risk nature of insulin and the impact of BG control on patient outcomes, careful care coordination throughout the continuum of care is needed for hospitalized patients using insulin. A dedicated inpatient diabetes management service following established standards of care improves results, stabilizes metabolic state, maintains stable glycemic levels, and facilitates a seamless transition to outpatient care with pre-scheduled follow-up appointments.[3] These efforts result in positive patient outcomes, shorter hospital stays, lower intensive care unit (ICU) time, and fewer emergency department visits and readmissions.[5] It is recommended that the team consisting of trained specialists in diabetes care establish comprehensive protocols for managing dysglycemia throughout all departments whether ICU or non-ICU units. These protocols should incorporate validated written or computerized provider order entry sets, allowing a personalized approach, which can improve workflow efficiency and minimize medication errors. The protocols should address BG monitoring, insulin and non-insulin therapy use, hypoglycemia management, diabetes self-management education and support (DSMES), nutrition recommendations, and care transitions.[5] The implementation of insulin order sets in one study resulted in a reduction of over 55% in potentially serious adverse events. Insulin order sets should be incorporated into electronic medical records to promote evidence-based prescribing.[36] Equally important is providing training to staff and conducting assessments on patients' DSMES knowledge and behaviors at the time of admission.[5]

Due to the risks of hypo and hyperglycemia, special attention must be paid to the management of diabetes medications during the transition from hospital to ambulatory care settings. Patient diets are often quite different post-discharge than they are inpatient. Conversations around meal preferences, timing, and food access should occur before mealtime insulin discharge instructions are established. For home medications, particularly non-insulin antihyperglycemic, intended to be restarted at discharge it is recommended to resume use 1 to 2 days prior to discharge.[5] This practice allows for the evaluation of BG control and adverse drug effects while still in a monitored setting.

Similarly, product interchanges are often implemented due to hospital formularies during inpatient stays. Before discharge, clarify with the patient which home medications are intended to be restarted or discontinued post-discharge. Ensuring the patient does not restart a home medication that duplicates a discharge medication (eg, 2 different basal insulin products) will prevent avoidable adverse events and readmissions. For patients on concentrated insulins prior to admission, clarification of product and dosing are especially important.

Given the variety of medications within each therapeutic class, verification of insurance coverage before discharge is crucial. The mean out-of-pocket cost per fill for insulin in patients without insurance is estimated to be $123.[37] Cost reduction strategies include patient assistance programs, sliding scale payment access through federally qualified health centers and safety net providers, and coupons.[37] Vials tend to have lower costs than pre-filled syringes.[18] Biosimilar follow-on products tend to have lower costs than reference products.[18] The Inflation Reduction Act of 2022 limits out-of-pocket costs for each insulin product to $35 per month for patients with Medicare coverage.[37] Insurance formularies should be consulted to identify preferred products for patients with non-Medicare insurance, though co-pays or co-insurances can still be expensive with some plans. Metformin, SUs, and TZDs are available as generic products, covered by most insurances, and included on many discount drug lists.[18] GLP1 RAs, GLP1 RA/GIPs, DPP4 inhibitors, and SGLT2 inhibitors are only available as brand products with median average wholesale price $161-1,072.[18] As coverage can vary significantly among plans, and out-of-pocket costs can be prohibitive, ensuring the patient has access to the medications on the discharge plan are critical to treatment success.

SUMMARY

Insulin is commonly used to mitigate the adverse outcomes of hyperglycemia in hospitalized patients. Evidence-based policies and protocols integrated into electronic health records for insulin and diabetes technologies improve the delivery of patient care. Shared decision-making and considerations of individualized patient factors are vital for hyperglycemic management, emphasizing the benefit of a multidisciplinary team with diabetes expertise.

CLINICS CARE POINTS

- Stress-induced hyperglycemia is common in hospitalized and critically ill patients.
- Insulin is the best way to control hyperglycemia in hospitalized patients. The blood glucose (BG) goals are 100-180 mg/dL for non-critically ill patients, 140-180 mg/dL for critically ill patients, and less than 250 mg/dL for terminally ill patients.
- There are a variety of insulin products that differ by concentration, route of administration, onset and duration of effect.
- Basal plus bolus insulin regimens are appropriate for many hospitalized patients. Doses need to be adjusted often due to BG values, diet, anticipated procedures, concomitant medications, and disease process.
- Patients with type 2 diabetes may also be on non-insulin antidiabetic agents. Many of these will be held during hospitalizations. Safety monitoring and confirmation of medication orders at transitions of care are important for safe use of these medications.
- Involvement of a diabetes specialty care team and establishment of protocols for managing dysglycemia throughout all departments, improve the care of patients with diabetes.

DISCLOSURES

The authors have nothing to disclose. Disclaimer: During the preparation of this work, the author(s) used Grammarly and Bing Chat Enterprise to improve readability and language of the work and not to replace key author tasks such as producing scientific, pedagogic, or medical insights, draw scientific conclusion or provide clinical recommendations. After using this tool/service, the author(s) reviewed and edited the content as needed and take(s) full responsibility for the content of the publication.

REFERENCES

1. Seisa MO, Saadi S, Nayfeh T, et al. A systematic review supporting the endocrine society clinical practice guideline for the management of hyperglycemia in adults hospitalized for noncritical illness or undergoing elective surgical procedures. J Clin Endocrinol Metab 2022;107(8):2139–47. Available at: https://pubmed.ncbi.nlm.nih.gov/35690929/.
2. Ma H, Yu G, Wang Z, et al. Association between dysglycemia and mortality by diabetes status and risk factors of dysglycemia in critically ill patients: a retrospective study. Acta Diabetol 2022;59(4):461–70. Available at: https://pubmed.ncbi.nlm.nih.gov/34761326/.
3. Sun H, Saeedi P, Karuranga S, et al. IDF Diabetes Atlas: global, regional, and country-level diabetes prevalence estimates for 2021 and projections for 2045. Diabetes Res Clin Pract 2022;183:109119.
4. Department of Health and Human Services. Centers for Medicare, and Medicaid Services (CMS). Subject: fiscal year (FY) 2009 inpatient prospective payment system (IPPS), long-term care hospital (LTCH) PPS, and inpatient psychiatric facility (IPF) PPS changes. Medicare claims processing. 2008. Available at: http://www.cms.hhs.gov/transmittals/downloads/R1610CP.pdf. [Accessed 6 April 2024].

5. American Diabetes Association Professional Practice Committee. Diabetes care in the hospital: standards of care in diabetes—2024. Diabetes Care 2024;47(Supp 1): S295–306. Available at: https://diabetesjournals.org/care/article/47/Supplement_ 1/S295/153950/16-Diabetes-Care-in-the-Hospital-Standards-of-Care.

6. Korytkowski MT, Muniyappa R, Antinori-Lent K, et al. Management of hyperglycemia in hospitalized adult patients in non-critical care settings: an endocrine society clinical practice guideline. J Clin Endocrinol Metab 2022 Jul 14;107(8): 2101–28. Available at: https://pubmed.ncbi.nlm.nih.gov/35690958/.

7. Honarmand K, Sirimaturos M, Hirshberg E, et al. Society of Critical Care Medicine guidelines on glycemic control for critically ill children and adults 2024. Crit Care Med 2024;52(4):e161–81. Online special article. Available at: https://pubmed. ncbi.nlm.nih.gov/38240484/.

8. NICE-SUGAR Study Investigators, Finfer S, Chittock DR, et al. Intensive versus conventional glucose control in critically ill patients. N Engl J Med 2009;360(13): 1283–97.

9. PharMerica corporation. Insulin – comparison chart. Available at: https://pharmerica. com/wp-content/uploads/2022/05/DidYouKnow_Insulin_Insulin-Comparison-Chart_ 04.2022.pdf. [Accessed 15 February 2024].

10. Riggs AD. Making, cloning and the expression of human insulin genes in bacteria: the path to Humulin. Endocr Rev 2021;42(3):374–80.

11. Bolli GB, Cheng AYY, Owens DR. Insulin: evolution of insulin formulations and their application in clinical practice over 100 years. Acta Diabetol 2022;59(9): 1129–44. Available at: https://www.ncbi.nlm.nih.gov/pmc/articles/PMC9296014/.

12. Hirsch IB, Juneja R, Beals JM, et al. The Evolution of insulin and how it informs therapy and treatment choices. Endocr Rev 2020;41(5):733–55. Available at: https://pubmed.ncbi.nlm.nih.gov/32396624/.

13. Tresiba (insulin degludec) injection, for subcutaneous use [package insert]. Plainsboro, NJ: Novo Nordisk Inc; 2022. Available at: https://www.accessdata.fda.gov/ drugsatfda_docs/label/2022/203314s018s020lbl.pdf. [Accessed 15 February 2024].

14. Kolanczyk DM, Dobersztyn RC. Challenges with insulin in the inpatient setting. Diabetes Spectr 2016;29(3):146–52.

15. Mehta R, Goldenberg R, Katselnik D, et al. Practical guidance on the initiation, titration, and switching of basal insulins: a narrative review for primary care. Ann Med 2021;53(1):999–1010. Available at: https://pubmed.ncbi.nlm.nih.gov/ 34165382/.

16. Pinnaro CT, Tansey MJ. The evolution of insulin administration in type 1 diabetes. J Diabetes Mellitus 2021 Nov;11(5):249–77. Available at: https://pubmed.ncbi. nlm.nih.gov/37745178/.

17. Afrezza (insulin human) inhalation powder [package insert]. Danbury, CT: Mannkind Corporation; 2023. Available at: https://afrezza.com/wp-content/uploads/ 2023/02/Full-Prescribing-Information-Feb-2023.pdf. [Accessed 1 April 2024].

18. American Diabetes Association Professional Practice Committee. Diabetes technology: standards of care in diabetes – 2024. Diabetes Care 2024;47(Suppl 1): S126–44.

19. Rushakoff RJ. Inpatient diabetes management. [Updated 2019 jan 7]. In: Feingold KR, Anawalt B, Blackman MR, et al, editors. Endotext Internet. South Dartmouth (MA): MDText.com, Inc; 2000. Available at: https://www.ncbi.nlm.nih. gov/books/NBK278972/.

20. Nau KC, Lorenzetti RC, Cucuzzella M, et al. Glycemic control in hospitalized patients not in intensive care: beyond sliding-scale insulin. Am Fam Physician 2010 May 1;81(9):1130–5. Available at: https://pubmed.ncbi.nlm.nih.gov/20433129/.
21. Lee YY, Lin YM, Leu WJ, et al. Sliding-scale insulin used for blood glucose control: a meta-analysis of randomized controlled trials. Metabolism 2015;64(9): 1183–92.
22. Gianchandani RY, Iyengar JL, Butler SO, et al. Inpatient diabetes guideline for adult non-critically ill patients [Internet]. Ann Arbor (MI): Michigan Medicine University of Michigan; 2020 May 22. Available at: https://pubmed.ncbi.nlm.nih.gov/32931166/.
23. Schnipper JL, Ndumele CD, Liang CL, et al. Effects of a subcutaneous insulin protocol, clinical education, and computerized order set on the quality of inpatient management of hyperglycemia: results of a clinical trial. J Hosp Med 2009;4(1):16–27.
24. Umpierrez GE, Hellman R, Korytkowski MT, et al. Management of hyperglycemia in hospitalized patients in non-critical care setting: an endocrine society clinical practice guideline. J Clin Endocrinol Metab 2012;97(1):16–38.
25. American diabetes association professional practice committee; 9. Pharmacologic approaches to glycemic treatment: standards of care in diabetes—2024. Diabetes Care 2024;47(Supplement_1):S158–78.
26. Preiser JC, Provenzano B, Mongkolpum W, et al. Perioperative management of oral glucose-lowering drugs in the patient with Type 2 Diabetes. Anesthesiology 2020;133:430–8. Available at: https://pubmed.ncbi.nlm.nih.gov/32667156/.
27. Joshi GP, Abdelmalak BB, Weigel WA, et al. American Society of Anesthesiologists Consensus-based guidance on preoperative management of patients (adults and children) on glucagon-like peptide-1 (GLP-1) receptor agonists. American Society of Anesthesiologists. Available at: https://www.asahq.org/about-asa/newsroom/news-releases/2023/06/american-society-of-anesthesiologists-consensus-based-guidance-on-preoperative. [Accessed 29 February 2024].
28. Dogra P, Anastasopoulou C, Jialal I. Diabetic perioperative management. StatPearls. 2024. Available at: https://pubmed.ncbi.nlm.nih.gov/31082009/. [Accessed 29 February 2024].
29. Cogle S, Hutchison AM, Mulherin DW. Finding the sweet spot: managing parenteral nutrition–related glycemic complications in hospitalized adults. Nutr Clin Pract 2023;38(6):1263–72. Available at: https://pubmed.ncbi.nlm.nih.gov/37749749/.
30. Jakoby MG, Nannapaneni N. An insulin protocol for management of hyperglycemia in patients receiving parenteral nutrition is superior to ad hoc management. JPEN J Parenter Enteral Nutr 2012;36(2):183–8.
31. Pancorbo-Hidalgo PL, Garcia-Fernandez FP, Ramirez-Perez C. Complications associated with enteral nutrition by nasogastric tube in an internal medicine unit. J Clin Nurs 2001 Jul;10(4):482–90.
32. Ayers P, Adams S, Boullata J, et al. American Society for Parenteral and Enteral Nutrition. A.S.P.E.N. parenteral nutrition safety consensus recommendations. JPEN J Parenter Enteral Nutr 2014;38(3):296–333.
33. McMahon MM. Management of parenteral nutrition in acutely ill patients with hyperglycemia. Nutr Clin Pract 2004;19:120–8.
34. Pasquel F, Lansang MC, Dhatariya K, et al. Management of diabetes and hyperglycemia in the hospital. Lancet Diabetes Endocrinol 2021;9:174–88.
35. The Joint Commission, Safe patient use of insulin pumps & CGM devices during hospitalization, Quick Safety, 59, 2021, 1–3, Available at: https://www.jointcommission.

org/resources/news-and-multimedia/newsletters/newsletters/quick-safety/quick-safety-issue-59/. (Accessed 6 April, 2024)

36. Sly B, Russell AW, Sullivan C. Digital interventions to improve safety and quality of inpatient diabetes management: a systematic review. Int J Med Inform 2022 Jan; 157:104596.

37. Sayed BA, Finegold K, Olsen A, et al. Insulin affordability and the inflation reduction act: Medicare beneficiary savings by state and demographics. (Issue brief No. HP-2023-02). Office of the assistant secretary for planning and evaluation, U.S. Department of health, and human services. 2023. Available at: https://aspe.hhs.gov/reports/insulin-affordability-ira-data-point. [Accessed 6 April 2024].

Perioperative Management of the Patient with Diabetes Mellitus

Celia Ann Levesque, APRN, NP-C, CNS-BC, CDCES, BC-ADM*

KEYWORDS

- Diabetes mellitus • Surgery • Perioperative • Anesthesia • Diabetes medications

KEY POINTS

- Patients with diabetes mellitus are at higher risk for adverse complications during the perioperative time.
- Half of all patients who have diabetes will have surgery during their lifetime.
- Patients with diabetes mellitus need careful evaluation prior to surgery to minimize risk for adverse complications related to surgery.
- Most diabetes medications need to be adjusted during the perioperative time.
- Management of blood glucose before, during, and after surgery is important to reduce the risk for hypoglycemia, extreme hyperglycemia, diabetic ketoacidosis, impaired wound healing, readmission, and prolonged length of stay.

INTRODUCTION

Approximately 38.4 million (11.6%) Americans have diabetes mellitus (DM)[1] and 8.4 million use insulin to treat DM.[2] Half of all patients with DM will have surgery in their lifetime and approximately 15% of patients undergoing surgery have DM. Each year approximately 64 million surgical procedures are performed. People with DM have a higher risk of postoperative complications compare to those without DM having the same operative procedure. Complications include delayed wound healing, infection, renal dysfunction, readmission, and longer length of stay.[3–5] Effective management of diabetes during the perioperative time involves an interdisciplinary team including, the surgical team, anesthesiology, endocrinology or internal medicine, nursing, and sometimes other specialists such as certified diabetes care and education specialists, dietitians, nephrologists, and cardiologists.

Department of Endocrine Neoplasia and Hormonal Disorders, The University of Texas MD Anderson Cancer Center, Houston, TX, USA
* Corresponding author. 1515 Holcomb Boulevard, Houston, TX 77030
E-mail address: clevesqu@mdanderson.org

Crit Care Nurs Clin N Am 37 (2025) 133–145
https://doi.org/10.1016/j.cnc.2024.05.003
ccnursing.theclinics.com
0899-5885/25/© 2024 Elsevier Inc. All rights reserved, including those for text and data mining, AI training, and similar technologies.

Surgery and anesthesia cause a neuroendocrine release of counterregulatory hormones including inflammatory cytokines (interleukin-6, and tumor necrosis factor-alpha), epinephrine, glucagon, cortisol, and growth hormone which can cause increased insulin resistance, proteolysis, and lipolysis, and decreased insulin secretion and uptake of glucose in peripheral tissue. These factors can lead to hyperglycemia and ketosis. Epidural or regional anesthesia does not impact blood glucose (BG) significantly.[6–9]

DISCUSSION

Prior to surgery, patients with DM need to have a detailed history, physical examination, laboratory testing, and additional testing as needed to evaluate comorbid conditions. A plan for adjusting DM medications needs to be given to the patient and a plan needs to be in place during and after surgery for managing BG while the patient is in the surgical facility or hospital. The patient also needs to be given a plan for managing DM after discharge.

HISTORY
Type of Diabetes Mellitus

Most patients with DM have type 1 diabetes (T1D) or type 2 diabetes (T2D). Some have other types of DM characterized by insulin deficiency or insulin resistance or varying degrees of both. T1D is an autoimmune destruction of beta cells leading to insulin deficiency as evidenced by low connecting peptide (C-peptide) and insulin therapy is required to prevent diabetic ketoacidosis (DKA) and death. T2D is characterized by progressive insulin resistance with beta cell failure. The patient may have high, normal, or low C-peptide. Some with T2D require insulin therapy to achieve glycemic targets and some are prone to DKA when under stress.[10] Other types of diabetes have a varying degree of insulin deficiency and/or insulin resistance and may be prone to development of DKA if under stress or insulin is omitted[11] (Table 1).

Duration of Diabetes Mellitus

The greater the duration of DM, the higher the risk for long-term DM-related complications and severe hypoglycemia. In patients with T2D, a longer duration may result in decreased insulin production and a higher risk of developing DKA.[12]

Hemoglobin A1c

The hemoglobin A1c (HbA1c) should be checked preoperative in all patients with DM unless there is a condition that renders the HbA1c inaccurate. Higher HbA1c levels are associated with worse outcomes such as wound infections, longer length of stay, and intensive care unit admission; however, there is no evidence that postponing surgery to improve BG control improves outcomes. Perioperative BG control has been shown to improve outcomes compared to HbA1c. If surgery is not urgent, and the HbA1c is over 8.5% or BG is over 250 mg/dL, elective surgery should be postponed until the glycemic control is achieved.[4,8,13]

Current Glycemic Control

Assess current BG control including history of frequency and severity of hypoglycemia and hypoglycemia unawareness. If the patient wears a continuous glucose monitor (CGM), assess the past 2-week report for time in range, time spent low, and variability. Ideally, the preoperative BG at the time of surgery should be less than 200 mg/dL.[13]

Table 1 Types and characteristics of diabetes mellitus	
Type of Diabetes	**Characteristics**
1	Autoimmune beta cell destruction leading to absolute insulin deficiency. Requires insulin to prevent diabetic ketoacidosis. • Typical type 1 diabetes • Latent autoimmune diabetes in adults • Immunotherapy-induced type 1 diabetes
2	Progressive insulin resistance with beta cell failure resulting in relative insulin deficiency. Usually occurs in adults but may occur in children. May require insulin treatment. Can develop diabetes-related ketoacidosis when under stress.
Gestational	Onset of diabetes that occurs during pregnancy. If diabetes remains after pregnancy, the diabetes is reclassified. Some patients require insulin therapy.
Monogenic diabetes syndromes	Diabetes secondary to genetic mutations • Neonatal diabetes with onset <6 mo. It may be transient or permanent and may require insulin therapy. • Maturity-onset diabetes of the young is characterized by impaired insulin secretion with little defect in insulin action in the absence of obesity.
Exocrine pancreatic disorders	Structural and functional loss of insulin secretion due to exocrine pancreatic dysfunction • Cystic fibrosis related diabetes • Pancreatitis (acute or chronic) • Pancreatic cancer • Trauma to the pancreas • Surgical removal (part or all) of the pancreas • Hemochromatosis • Fibrocalculous pancreatopathy • Rare genetic disorders • Idiopathic forms
Medication-induced	Medications that impair insulin secretion, insulin action, or both. Common drug classes causing hyperglycemia include the following (not a complete list): • Glucocorticoids • Phosphoinositide 3-kinase inhibitors • Immunosuppression drugs • Antipsychotics • Antiretrovirals

Presence of Diabetes Mellitus–Related Acute and Chronic Complications and Comorbid Conditions

Patients with DM are at higher risk for diabetes-related kidney disease, peripheral and autonomic neuropathy, diabetes-related retinopathy, coronary artery disease, silent ischemia, cerebrovascular disease, peripheral vascular disease, hypertension, and after surgery, venous thromboembolism, and bleeding. Assess for a previous history of DKA, hospitalization for hyperglycemia, and hyperosmolar hyperglycemic state. Optimize comorbid conditions if possible before surgery.[4,7]

Age of the Patient

Advanced age, in general, conveys a higher risk for surgery. Older patients have a higher rate of comorbid conditions.[7]

Urgency, Type, and Duration of Surgery

The classifications for urgency of surgery include emergency (within 6 hours), urgent (within 24 hours), time-sensitive (1–6 weeks), and elective (up to 1 year). If the surgery is elective and the diabetes control is not optimized, then surgery should be postponed until glycemic targets are achieved. The type of surgery varies considerably and the risk for complications depends on many factors including the location, depth of surgery within the tissue, blood loss, and fluid shifts. The more extensive surgery and the longer duration in surgery under anesthesia can increase risk for complications.[7]

Nutrition Before and After Surgery

Assess the amount of time that the patient will be on a clear-liquid diet before surgery, the amount of time the patient will be nothing by mouth (NPO) before and after surgery, and what type of diet the patient will be on after surgery. When the patient is on a clear-liquid diet, the patient may consume clear liquids without carbohydrate to prevent dehydration or with carbohydrate to prevent ketosis and prevent or treat hypoglycemia. If the patient uses insulin and the BG is not low, prandial insulin can be used to treat clear-liquid carbohydrate. If the patient will be NPO for a prolonged period after surgery, then intravenous (IV) dextrose, enteral nutrition, or parenteral nutrition may be needed depending on the amount of time the patient will be NPO, the current nutritional status, and nutritional needs of the patient.

TESTING BEFORE SURGERY

- Kidney function tests
- HbA1c
- BG
- Electrocardiogram
- If indicated
  - Cardiac stress testing
  - Echocardiography
  - B-natriuretic peptide
  - Other tests as indicated based on history and physical examination. Assessment tools for assessing risk of venous thromboembolism and bleeding may need to be utilized.[7]

GLYCEMIC GOALS FOR SURGERY

Glycemic goals for most patients with DM undergoing surgery is 110 to 180 mg/dL but the goal may need to adjusted depending on the patient's circumstances including age, the risk of hypoglycemia, comorbid conditions, life expectancy, and renal and liver function. If the patient is taking a sulfonylureas (SU), meglitinides, or insulin, then the desired BG is over 100 mg/dL before surgery.[8,9,14]

FREQUENCY OF GLUCOSE TESTING

The BG is usually tested every 2 hours in the presurgery and postsurgery area. During surgery, the BG is usually tested every 2 hours if insulin is being given subcutaneously and every 1 hour if the patient is receiving an insulin drip.[13,15]

TIMING OF SURGERY

Ideally, surgery should be in the morning if possible.

DIABETES MEDICATION REGIMEN

Assess the names, dose, and frequency of DM medications. If the patient is taking insulin, SU, or meglitinides, assess to see if the patient develops hypoglycemia when missing a meal. If the patient uses an insulin pump, assess their knowledge in programming and caring for their insulin pump.

ADJUSTMENT OF NON-INSULIN DIABETES MEDICATIONS FOR SURGERY
Sodium-Glucose Cotransporter 2 Inhibitors

Sodium-glucose cotransporter 2 inhibitors (SGLT-2is) are commonly used to treat T2D, heart failure (HF), and to slow the progression of chronic kidney disease (CKD). This drug class increases the risk of euglycemic DKA (eDKA) which is defined at pH less than 7.3, bicarbonate less than 15 mmol/L, BG less than 252 mg/dL, and anion gap greater than 12. SGLT-2is reduce renal threshold for spilling glucose into the urine from approximately 180 mg/dL to 70 to 90 mg/dL, thus causing glycosuria and reduced BG. The reduced BG causes the pancreas to increase glucagon and decrease insulin production which leads to increased lipolysis, ketone formation, and free fatty acids, thus increasing the risk for eDKA.

Risk factors for SGLT-2i-induced eDKA during the perioperative time:

- Procedure greater than 1 hour
- General anesthesia
- HbA1c over 8% before surgery
- BG over 150 mg/dL before surgery
- Patients requiring insulin before surgery/reduced insulin dose.
- DM with comorbid conditions
- Fever/illness
- NPO greater than 12 hours or reduced food intake for prolonged period

Relative insulin deficiency combined with decreased carbohydrate intake causes increased levels of glucagon and catecholamines leading to lipolysis and increased ketones potentially leading to eDKA; however, since the BG levels are lower than expected in DKA due to glycosuria, it is often not recognized early in eDKA. The Food and Drug Administration in May 2020 began recommending that SGLT-2is be held 3 to 4 days prior to surgery, depending on the brand (**Tables 2–4**).

For those who have held the SGLT-2is according to recommendations do not need additional laboratory testing except BG on the day of surgery but if carbohydrate intake is not resumed within 2 hours after surgery, a basic metabolic panel (BMP) is needed to screen for eDKA and the BMP needs to be repeated every 12 hours until the patient is consuming carbohydrate. If the patient did not hold the SGLT-2i according to recommendations, the patient needs to be screened for eDKA with a BMP to calculate anion gap and β-hydroxybutyrate (BOHB). If the anion gap is greater than 12, surgery should be postponed. If surgery is not postponed, then within 1 hour after surgery the BG, BMP, and serum BOHB should be measured, and hyperglycemia treated. The BMP and BOHB should be checked again 4 hours after surgery then every 8 hours for the first 24 hours. After the first 24 hours, check BMP every 12 hours if tolerating a diet and add BOHB if still NPO. If any BMP shows bicarbonate 18 or less, a pH less than 7.3, or calculated anion gap of 12 or higher, check BOHB and serum lactate. Consider dextrose IV if the patient will be NPO after the procedure and give insulin subcutaneously or via IV if needed. If the patient has T1D and was using an SGLT-2is for HF or CKD, then basal insulin is needed to prevent eDKA, prandial insulin is needed for carbohydrate, and correctional insulin is needed to correct

Table 2
Non-insulin diabetes medications for surgery

Diabetes Medication Class	Before Surgery	Day of Surgery	After Surgery
SGLT-2is	Hold 3 d before • Bexagliflozin • Canagliflozin • Dapagliflozin • Empagliflozin Hold 4 d before • Ertugliflozin	Hold all SGLT-2is	Resume if eating and drinking well and no contraindications.
GLP-1 RA and dual GLP-1 RA and GIP	Daily GLP-1: Hold for 1 d before surgery. Weekly GLP-1 RA and dual GLP-1 RA and GIP: Hold for 1 wk before surgery	Hold	Resume if eating well and no contraindications
Metformin	Continue	Hold	Resume if no contraindication
Sulfonylureas or meglitinides	Consider reducing or holding the dose if prone to hypoglycemia and if not eating usual amounts of food	Hold	Resume if eating well and no contraindications
Thiazolidinediones	Continue	Hold	Resume if no contraindications
Alpha-glucosidase inhibitor	Continue if eating meals	Hold	Resume if eating well and no contraindications
Dipeptidyl peptidase-4 inhibitor	Continue	Hold	Resume if no contraindications
Amylin Agonist	Continue if eating meals	Hold	Resume if eating well and no contraindications

Table 3
Adjustment of insulin in patients with type 2 diabetes for surgery[8,13]

Insulin Regimen	Day before Surgery	Day of Surgery	After Surgery
Basal insulin once daily No rapid-acting/short-acting insulin	May need to reduce dose if eating less than usual or prolonged fasting causes hypoglycemia	May need to reduce or hold until after surgery	Resume basal insulin, the dose depends on nutrition intake and BG levels.
Basal insulin twice daily	May need to reduce dose if eating less than usual or prolonged fasting causes hypoglycemia	May need to reduce or hold until after surgery	Resume basal insulin, the dose depends on nutrition intake and BG levels.
Basal insulin with prandial/correctional insulin	May need to reduce dose if eating less than usual or prolonged fasting causes hypoglycemia. Take prandial/correctional insulin as usual for meals and treatment of hyperglycemia	May need to reduce or hold until after surgery. Prandial insulin is held until the patient resumes eating. Correctional insulin is given by nursing/anesthesia while the patient is in the preop, surgery, and postop area	Resume basal insulin with prandial/correctional insulin, the doses dependent on nutrition intake and BG levels.
Premixed insulin twice daily	The evening dose is often reduced the evening before surgery	One-half of the usual morning dose is given as NPH. If the morning BG is > 200 mg/dL then one-half of the premixed insulin is given	Resume premixed insulin; the dose depends on nutrition intake and BG levels
Insulin pump	Continue using usual doses. May need to reduce basal rate if prolonged fasting causes hypoglycemia.	The patient may be required to suspend delivery or remove pump for surgery. The patient may receive basal and or correctional insulin during surgery.	Resume insulin pump once awake and alert and able operate. Doses may need to be adjusted after surgery.

Table 4
Adjustment of insulin for surgery in patients with type 1 diabetes and any patient with low connecting peptide

Insulin Regimen	Day before Surgery	Day of Surgery	After Surgery
Basal with prandial and correctional insulin	Take usual doses. May need reduced basal dose if prolonged fasting causes hypoglycemia	Give usual basal dose. May need reduced dose if prolonged fasting causes hypoglycemia. Prandial insulin is held until the patient is eating after surgery. Give correctional insulin subcutaneous for hyperglycemia every 2–4 h or IV insulin infusion	Give usual basal dose unless prolonged fasting causes hypoglycemia. Give prandial insulin for food consumed. Give correctional insulin to treat hyperglycemia every 2–4 h. If on IV insulin infusion during surgery, do not abruptly stop unless basal insulin has been given before discontinuation of IV insulin infusion.

hyperglycemia. If the patient is being discharged the same day as the procedure, the patient needs to be able to tolerate nutrition and the BG levels should be less than 150 mg/dL prior to discharge.

SGLT-2is can be restarted the day after surgery if the patient is able to tolerate nutrition and there are no contraindications. The patient should be instructed to seek medical attention if nausea, vomiting, confusion, inability to tolerate nutrition, or BG is over 250 mg/dL[4,16,17] (**Fig. 1**).

Glucagon-like-Peptide 1 Receptor Agonists and Dual Glucagon-like-Peptide 1 Receptor Agonists with Gastric Inhibitory Polypeptide Receptor Agonists

Glucagon-like-peptide 1 receptor agonists (GLP-1 RAs) and dual GLP-1 RAs with gastric inhibitory polypeptide (GIP) receptor agonists delay gastric emptying, increasing the risk for pulmonary aspiration, so the daily GLP-1 RA medications should be held 1 day before surgery and the weekly GLP-1 RA and dual GLP-1 RA and GIP should be held 1 week before surgery[4,16,18] (See **Table 2**).

Metformin

Metformin is the most prescribed medication for T2D. It should not be used in any medical condition that carries increased risk for lactic acidosis such as CKD, liver disease, and HF. If the estimated glomerular filtration rate is less than 45, metformin should not be started in patients who are not already on metformin, and if less than 30, it should be discontinued. Metformin should be held on the day of surgery and resumed after surgery if there are no contraindications such as impaired renal function or lactic acidosis (see **Table 2**).[4,16]

Sulfonylureas and Meglitinides

SU and meglitinides (glinide) cause insulin secretion by closing ATP-sensitive potassium channels on the beta cell plasma membrane. The most common side effect is hypoglycemia, especially if the patient has reduced nutritional intake. If the patient is eating usual amounts the day before surgery, then the patient can take them. SU

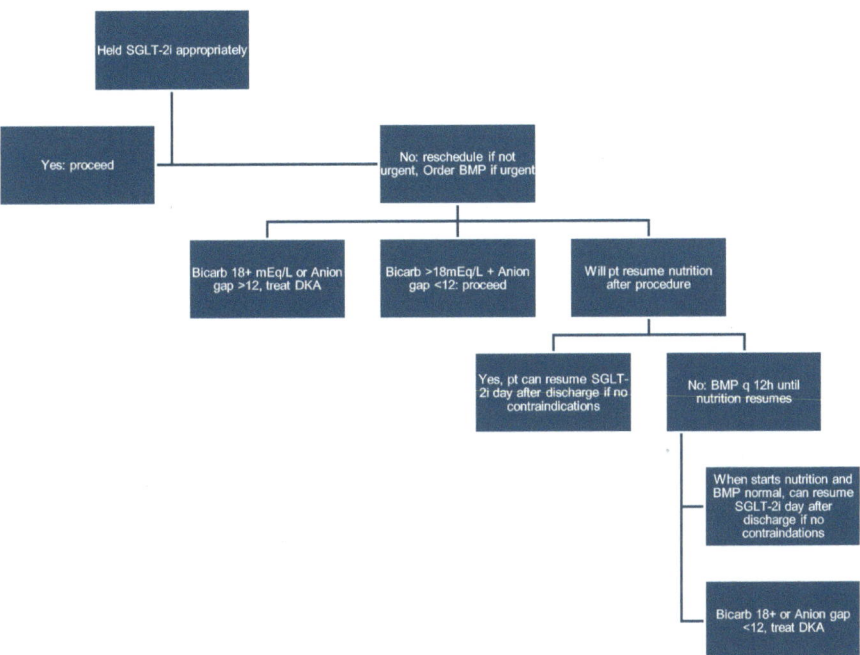

Fig. 1. Decision tree for sodium-glucose cotransporter 2 inhibitors in the perioperative setting.

and meglitinides need to be held the day of surgery and only resumed once the patient has adequate nutritional intake. Since SU work for 1 to 3 days, then some patients may need to reduce or hold SU the day before surgery (see **Table 2**).[4,16]

Thiazolidinediones

Thiazolidinediones activate nuclear transcription factor PPAR-alpha, increasing sensitivity and decreasing hepatic gluconeogenesis. It is contraindicated in New York HF classes III and IV. It can be taken the day before surgery, held the day of surgery, and resumed after surgery if there are no contraindications[4,16] (see **Table 2**).

Alpha-glucosidase Inhibitors

Alpha-glucosidase inhibitors (AGIs) block intestinal alpha-glucosidase inhibiting absorption of glucose from the intestine. They are contraindicated in patients with any intestinal disease or obstruction, and cirrhosis. They are taken with meals so if the patient is eating the day before surgery, the medication can be given but held on the day of surgery and not resumed until the patient is eating well and has no contraindications. If a patient has hypoglycemia while taking an AGI, then only dextrose (not sucrose) can be used to treat.[16]

Dipeptidyl Peptidase-4 Inhibitor

Dipeptidyl peptidase-4 inhibitor inhibits DP-4 activity, increasing GLP-1 and GIP concentrations causing glucose-dependent insulin secretion. They do not cause hypoglycemia so the medication can be continued the day before surgery, held on the day of surgery, and resumed after surgery if there are no contraindications.[16]

Amylin Agonist

Amylin agonist is a synthetic analogue of the polypeptide pancreatic hormone amylin which slows gastric emptying, suppresses glucagon, and regulates appetite. If the patient is eating as usual the day before surgery, then it may be given. It needs to be held on the day of surgery and can be resumed after surgery if the patient is eating as usual if no contraindications.[16]

INSULIN PUMP DURING THE PERIOPERATIVE PERIOD

An insulin pump can be used by any patient with DM requiring insulin. Insulin pumps, except for patch insulin pumps, are programmed by the user to deliver a continuous basal rate used to maintain normoglycemia between meals, and a bolus rate to treat food and to correct hyperglycemia. Some brands are semiautomated in that the pump adjust basal rates and may deliver correctional doses for hyperglycemia based on CGM data from a compatible CGM. Two patch insulin pumps are currently on the US market: the V-Go which delivers a single basal rate that cannot be adjusted and delivers a 2-unit bolus increments with each button push to treat food and/or hyperglycemia, and the CeQur which is a bolus-only patch pump that delivers a 2-unit bolus increments with each button push. All insulin pumps use either short-acting or rapid-acting insulin. Most institutions have an insulin pump policy. Often, the policy has the patient wear the insulin pump to the surgery and then disconnect the insulin pump just prior to the start of the surgery, and resume once the patient is awake and alert. Some surgeons/anesthesiologists may allow the patient to wear the pump during surgery if the surgery is of short duration. If worn during surgery, then the patient may be asked to suspend insulin delivery during the surgery and resume delivery after surgery once the patient is awake and alert.[4,14]

INTRAVENOUS INSULIN INFUSION DURING SURGERY

IV insulin infusion requires frequent BG monitoring (usually every 1 hour), and adjustment based on current BG and rate of rise or fall from the previous BG level. A separate infusion of dextrose should be used. Close monitoring of potassium and bicarbonate is required. If IV insulin infusion is used during surgery, it should not be abruptly stopped after surgery until the patient has basal insulin on board. A basal-bolus insulin regimen, once IV insulin infusion is discontinued, has been shown to be more effective than the prolonged use of a sliding scale insulin regimen.[15,19,20]

HYPOGLYCEMIA WHILE AT SURGICAL FACILITY: PREOPERATIVELY, INTRAOPERATIVELY, AND POSTOPERATIVELY

Hypoglycemia is defined as a BG 70 mg/dL or less. Treatment of hypoglycemia is to stop insulin delivery, by administration of 25 mL IV dextrose 50% and repeating BG every 15 to 30 minutes and repeat treatment as needed.
  Risk factors for hypoglycemia include.

- Patients taking insulin, SU, or meglitinides
- Age over 70 years
- Malnourished
- Decreased renal or liver function.
- History of hypoglycemia
- Hypoglycemia unawareness
- Duration of DM

- Adrenal insufficiency
- Interruption of enteral or parenteral nutrition
- Alcohol intake[4,14]

POSTOPERATIVE GLYCEMIC MANAGEMENT

In patients using insulin therapy before surgery, if the patient has a basal and/or prandial insulin requirement, it is important to avoid ordering only sliding scale rapid-acting or short-acting insulin to correct hyperglycemia. If the patient is not eating, then basal and correctional insulin can be ordered initially and then prandial can be added once the patient begins to eat. If a patient did not need insulin prior to surgery, then it may be appropriate to begin with correctional insulin only, but if the patient is having hyperglycemia after surgery requiring correctional insulin, then the patient should be ordered basal and/or prandial insulin in addition to the correctional scale.[20]

SUMMARY

Management of diabetes during the perioperative time requires a comprehensive assessment, optimization of glycemic control, management of comorbid conditions, and adjustment of diabetes medications immediately before, during, and after surgery. Successful management requires a multidisciplinary approach with clear communication working toward a common goal of minimizing risk of postoperative complications in the patient with diabetes. Glucose control during the perioperative period is important to reduce the risk of postoperative complications.

CLINICS CARE POINTS

- Optimization of glucose and comorbid conditions is vital to minimize perioperative adverse events and outcomes.
- A thorough history, examination, and testing should be done prior to surgery for the patient with diabetes.
- A multidisciplinary approach should include the surgeon, anesthesia, the provider managing diabetes, and other providers if needed, such as those managing comorbid conditions, diabetes care and education specialists, and dietitians.
- Diabetes medications need to be adjusted appropriately before, during, and after surgery.
- BG needs to be monitored closely throughout the perioperative time period.
- Hypoglycemia needs to be avoided, and recognized and treated appropriately should it occur.
- Patients with T1D, low C-peptide, or high risk for DKA need to receive basal insulin to prevent DKA. Basal doses may need to be reduced if fasting for a prolonged period, but it should never be omitted. The patient will need short-acting or rapid-acting insulin to treat food and correct hyperglycemia.
- If IV insulin infusion is used during surgery, it should not be abruptly stopped without basal insulin on board.
- Patients using SGLT-2is need to hold for 3 to 4 days depending on the brand before surgery to reduce risk for eDKA.
- Patients using GLP-1 RA or dual GLP-1 RA and GIP need to hold 1 week before surgery if on a weekly injection, and 1 day before surgery if on a daily GLP-1 RA to reduce risk for aspiration.

- If insulin is needed after surgery, basal/prandial/correctional insulin regimens are more effective than sliding scale–only regimens.
- Avoid prolonged fasting in patients with diabetes. It increases the risk for hypoglycemia and ketoacidosis.
- Diabetes medication regimens may need to be adjusted at discharge. The patient needs to be instructed on the diabetes medication recommendations at discharge

DISCLOSURE

The author does not have any conflicts of interest to disclose.

REFERENCES

1. Centers for Disease Control and Prevention. National diabetes statistics report. Available at: https://www.cdc.gov/diabetes/data/statistics-report/index.html. [Accessed 2 May 2024].
2. American Diabetes Association. American diabetes association announces support for INSULIN act at senate press conference. Available at: https://diabetes.org/newsroom/american-diabetes-association-announces-support-for-insulin-act-at-senate-press-conference. [Accessed 2 May 2024].
3. Drayton DJ, Birch RJ, D'Souza-Ferrer C, et al. Diabetes mellitus and perioperative outcomes: a scoping review of the literature. Br J Anaesth 2022;128(5):817–28.
4. Duggan E, Chen Y. Glycemic management in the operating room: screening, monitoring, oral hypoglycemics, and insulin therapy. Curr Diabetes Rep 2019;19:1–13.
5. Rayman G, Page E, Hodgson S, et al. Improving the outcomes for people with diabetes undergoing surgery: an observational study of the Improving the Perioperative Pathway of People with Diabetes (IP3D) intervention. Diabetes Res Clin Pract 2024;207:111062.
6. Mahmoodiyeh B, Etemadi S, Kamali A, et al. Evaluating the effect of different types of anesthesia on intraoperative blood glucose levels in diabetics and non-diabetics patients: a systematic review and meta-analysis. Annals of the Romanian Society for Cell Biology 2021;2559–72.
7. Bierle DM, Raslau D, Regan DW, et al. Preoperative evaluation before noncardiac surgery. In Mayo Clinic Proceedings, Vol. 95, No. 4, 2020, Elsevier; Amsterdam, Netherlands. 807-822.
8. Vogt AP, Bally L. Perioperative glucose management: current status and future directions. Best Pract Res Clin Anaesthesiol 2020;34(2):213–24.
9. Sudhakaran S, Surani SR. Guidelines for perioperative management of the diabetic patient. Surgery research and practice 2015;2015:284063.
10. Kovacs A, Bunduc S, Veres DS, et al. One third of cases of new-onset diabetic ketosis in adults are associated with ketosis-prone type 2 diabetes—a systematic review and meta-analysis. Diabetes Metabol Res Rev 2024;40(3):e3743.
11. American Diabetes Association. 2. Diagnosis and classification of diabetes: standards of care in diabetes—2024. Diabetes Care 2024;47(Supplement_1):S20–42.
12. Ikegami H, Babaya N, Noso S. β-Cell failure in diabetes: common susceptibility and mechanisms shared between type 1 and type 2 diabetes. Journal of Diabetes Investigation 2021;12(9):1526–39.
13. Simha V, Shah P. Perioperative glucose control in patients with diabetes undergoing elective surgery. JAMA 2019;321(4):399–400.

14. Palermo NE, Garg R. Perioperative management of diabetes mellitus: novel approaches. Curr Diabetes Rep 2019;19:1–7.
15. Galway U, Chahar P, Schmidt MT, et al. Perioperative challenges in management of diabetic patients undergoing non-cardiac surgery. World J Diabetes 2021; 12(8):1255.
16. Preiser J-C, Provenzano B, Mongkolpun W, et al. Perioperative management of oral glucose-lowering drugs in the patient with type 2 diabetes. Anesthesiology 2020;133(2):430–8.
17. Raiten JM, Morlok A, D'Ambrosia S, et al. Perioperative management of patients receiving sodium-glucose cotransporter 2 inhibitors: development of a clinical guideline at a large academic medical center. J Cardiothorac Vasc Anesth 2024; 38(1):57–66.
18. Joshi GP. Anesthetic considerations in adult patients on glucagon-like peptide-1 receptor agonists: gastrointestinal focus. Anesth Analg 2022;10:1213.
19. Cheisson G, Jacqueminet S, Cosson E, et al. Perioperative management of adult diabetic patients. Intraoperative period. Anaesthesia Critical Care & Pain Medicine 2018;37:S21–5.
20. Pérez A, Ramos A, Carreras G. Insulin therapy in hospitalized patients. Am J Therapeut 2020;27(1):e71–8.

Diabetes Education for the Hospitalized Patient

Denise Ann Palma, MS, MBA, MHA, RD, LD, CDCES, BC-ADM

KEYWORDS

- Diabetes • Diabetes educator • Diabetes education • Hyperglycemia

KEY POINTS

- Diabetes education is a key component to safely discharge a patient when there is a change in status or newly diagnosed.
- Incorporating diabetes education into everyday bedside care can aid a person with diabetes (PWD) in building on the ADCES7 Self-Care Behaviors.
- A team approach in providing "survival skills" diabetes education is ideal to enable a safe discharge.
- Patient education is the foundation of good nursing practice and routine care.
- A health care organization should make best use of staff skills to provide brief but targeted diabetes education.

INTRODUCTION

Diabetes accounts for 25% of noncritically ill hospitalized adult patients in addition to other hospitalized patients experiencing hyperglycemia (blood glucose >140 mg/dL).[1] Diabetes and hyperglycemia are both associated with prolonged length of stay and increased incidence of complications.[1] In 2022, it was estimated that 25.5 million people in the United States had diagnosed diabetes representing 7.6% of the total population.[2] The estimated national cost of diabetes in 2022 was $412.9 billion, of which $306.6 billion (74%) represented direct health care expenditures due to diabetes and $106.3 billion (26%) represented lost productivity from work-related absenteeism, reduced productivity at work and at home, unemployment from chronic disability, and premature mortality.[2] Diabetes is a chronic disease requiring a person with diabetes (PWD) to make daily and perform self-management decisions.[3] DSME/S establishes a foundation to aid PWD navigate daily activities which as shown to improve health outcomes.[3] Diabetes self-management education (DSME) is the process of conducting the knowledge and skill necessary for diabetes self-care and diabetes self-management support (DSMS) refers the necessary foundation to sustain coping

Department of Endocrine Neoplasia and Hormonal Disorders, The University of Texas MD Anderson Cancer Center, 1515 Holcombe Boulevard, Houston, TX 77030, USA
E-mail address: dapalma@mdanderson.org

Crit Care Nurs Clin N Am 37 (2025) 147–155
https://doi.org/10.1016/j.cnc.2024.08.003
ccnursing.theclinics.com
0899-5885/25/© 2024 Elsevier Inc. All rights reserved, including those for text and data mining, AI training, and similar technologies.

skills and continue behavior to self-manage diabetes.[3] Diabetes education should be delivered to meet the patient's health care beliefs, cultural needs, knowledge base, physical impairments, emotional concerns, support systems, financial status, and other factors that may influence a PWD's ability to conduct self-management.[3] Diabetes self-management education and support (DSME/S) has demonstrated to be cost-effective by reducing hospital admissions and readmissions.[3] DSME/S aids the reduction of onset or progression of diabetes complications, improve quality of life, increase healthy coping and engage in physical activity.[3] The diabetes education algorithm provides an evidence-based method of identifying and referring PWD's to DSME/S.[3] The algorithm identifies 4 critical times to deliver key information on the self-management skills necessary for each critical point.[3] The 4 critical times to assess, provide, and adjust DSME/S: (1) new diagnosis, (2) annually for maintenance and prevention of complications, (3) when new complicating factors influence self-management, and (4) transition of care.[3] All providers should discuss with PWD's the benefits and value of initial and continued DSME/S.[4] Initial diabetes education introduction by health care teams can decrease fear and distress associated with newly diagnosed or ongoing care. Each provider included in daily contact with patients during hospital stay has an opportunity to encourage and reassure patient diabetes can be managed.

WHO

Newly diagnosed patients during inpatient stay can often be overwhelmed with fear, anger, myths along with life circumstances influencing acceptance.[4] Providers and nurses should set the stage when delivering initial care by taking the time to listen, provide emotional support by answering questions in order to develop a person-centered treatment plan.[4] Another opportunity can exist if patient is not meeting diabetes treatment targets which may benefit from review and reinforcement of treatment goals. Building rapport during inpatient stay can also uncover barriers to self-care which could be addressed before discharge. For example, a patient may need a medication refill or be unable to afford the current diabetes management plan. Health care providers should be careful to avoid implicit bias by carefully listening to patient needs. Patients may benefit from new techniques, technology and updated information to improve implementation of diabetes therapy. Health-literacy is known to be associated with the health outcomes of diabetes.[5] The term health-literacy refers to the capacity to obtain, process, and understand basic health information and services needed to make appropriate health decisions.[5] When delivering diabetes education a one-size fits all approach should be avoided as healthy literacy differs and different levels may exist in how patient accepts and navigates new information. A step-by-step and individualized approach may be more effective than information overload given in one session. Diabetes education is given over a series of encounters by all health care team members to reduce anxiety and build trust. Providing personal experiences should be avoided. A patient may experience a change or new complicating factor influencing their ability to manage glucose control. For example, a patient may initiate steroid treatment as part of cancer treatment causing significant changes to their plan of care. The patient should be assured diabetes management can change and they are not doing anything wrong. Reassuring the patient by providing appropriate resources and referrals to improve glucose levels. A transition of care may require a change in diabetes management plan which gives another opportunity to provide diabetes education. For example, patients may not be able to provide self-care temporarily or indefinitely and support systems will need diabetes education for at home care. Support systems also need assurance diabetes can be managed with proper training and resources. Become a leader by staying up to date on diabetes education and developing teaching skills to identify the who, what, when, where and why.[6] For example, a simple act incorporated in daily activities of bedside care can include thoroughly explaining how and why premeal insulin is injected to reduce the fear of injections. Patient experience during inpatient stay often creates a distorted realization of needles if completed improperly leading to unwanted fear and unnecessary discomfort. Take each opportunity to deliver quality care and education to reduce the fear and anxiety often associated with diabetes care.

WHAT

A framework provides guidance for DSME/S teams to utilize teaching strategies, and methods for evaluating learning outcomes when completing diabetes education.[7] The ADCES7 Self-Care Behaviors is an evidenced-based framework and outline to provide education on healthy coping, healthy eating, being active, taking medication, monitoring, reducing risk, problem solving.[7] The Association for Diabetes Care & Education's ADCES7 Self-Care Behaviors provide a model for assessment, intervention and evaluation for PWD's.[8]

Healthy coping is the core of the behaviors as it is defined as a positive attitude toward diabetes and self-management along with positive relationships with others and impact on quality of life.[8] Health care providers should aim to establish a patient-centered approach to reduce diabetes-related distress. Diabetes-related distress can be described as having an emotional burden of diabetes along with constant demands for daily self-management care which can heighten with lack of access to care and developing long-term complications.[8] PWD's are also prone to have or develop anxiety, depression, disordered eating and cognitive impairment.[8] Developing a relationship and rapport with a patient is key. Remember a PWD may be dealing with other factors in their daily life; diabetes may not be the priority. Develop and train how to conduct motivational interviewing by asking open ended questions to gain more insight into the patient's perspective. For example, a patient may be dealing with cancer treatment and glucose values may not be at goal. Instead of giving the patient a lecture on diabetes, attempt to understand their daily ability to implement care and access to support systems. Many times patients are treated as though being not compliant with recommendations is due to ignorance of the disease. Which is not true. Diabetes education allows the time to break it down and explain. PWD's simply want to understand the why. Diabetes management plans should be tailored to the patient's needs and abilities with the aim to slowly push toward the greater goal. Healthy coping allows us to build trust in order to move toward the other 6 behaviors.

Healthy eating can be influenced by several factors such as food and cultural preferences, food security, health beliefs and eating habits.[8] Healthy eating refers to the pattern of eating a wide variety of high-quality foods in portions that promote prime health and wellness.[8] The major challenge with healthy eating is ambiguity. A hospitalized patient may achieve glucose targets in a controlled environment with tailored meal plan and diet order. The hospital menu may also offer macronutrient description to assist meal selection and insulin dosing if warranted. A PWD may also have their sugary beverages limited by hospital staff. The patient must be informed of changes and understand the importance of dietary changes to aid glucose control. The changes must also be patient-centered and reasonable. For example, making extreme changes to diet which are not aligned with a patient's normal routine creates unrealistic expectations and goals. A patient-centered goal will take into consideration what the patient finds to be reasonable and potentially capable of transitioning dietary changes to daily routine upon discharge. Another example, the PWD may be a shift worker or does not cook. The patient will need assistance and guidance on how to navigate barriers and establish a best case scenario to implement their diabetes management plan of care. It's also essential to avoid using fear tactics or identifying foods as "forbidden foods". Again the aim is to help patients build skills to make the best selection of foods to promote prime wellness. The patient may benefit from understanding how to read a food label or identifying foods which impact glucose the most. Diabetes education serves as a motivator to build patient confidence in managing diabetes. Healthy eating is not giving a patient meal plan or telling them what to eat. Healthy eating is developing skills over time to tweak their current food selection into quality and reasonable selections. Examples of behaviors that contribute to healthier food selection: carbohydrates counting, the plate method, measure portions and monitor intake, understand and use the nutrition facts label.[8]

Being active may include all types, duration and intensities of daily physical movement contributing the bursts of aerobic or resistance training.[8] Discussing the importance of physical activity during hospital stay may be introduced as the benefits associated to cardiometabolic health.[8] A patient with higher cardiometabolic risk may need medical clearance and explore which types of physical activity are best suited for current condition.[8]

Taking medication behaviors include the following daily recommendations of prescribed treatment with respect to understanding dosing, timing and frequency.[8] Medication adherence is a crucial component in the prevention and management of chronic disease.[8] In addition, therapeutic interia, insufficient treatment interventions and skipping/missing medication are multifactorial.[8] Health care providers need to probe further before making conclusions as to why patient is not taking medication. A patient may be having difficulty filling the prescription due to transportation, access to care, or financial burden. Patients may also be experiencing common side effects associated with medication classification. Health and cultural beliefs about plan of care is an important discussion point when developing diabetes treatment plan.[8] For example, insulin carries a stigma with the perception of having the worst type of diabetes. Oftentimes, insulin is the quickest method to resolve hyperglycemia and patients should be given diabetes education on what insulin is. Some patients carry a negative memory of loved ones using insulin and daily injections; patients deserve the time and attention to share decision making around medication use which enhances engagement and improves outcomes.[8] Some common barriers reported include regimen complexity, adverse effects, remembering to take medication or obtaining refills, fear of insulin, mental health and patient's lack of belief in the benefits of the medication.[9]

Monitoring glucose has evolved with the use of continuous glucose monitoring (CGM). A patient may continue to utilize glucometer at home to complete fingersticks which continues to serve great purpose where technology is not available or accessible. The use of glucose monitoring is gathering data for pattern management but most importantly aid patients in decision making and accountability. Patients need to be given diabetes education on glucose ranges and ideal times to monitor. Hospitalized patients may voice their fear of needles during point of care (POC) glucose monitoring; hospital staff should utilize this opportunity to reduce fear by acknowledging their concerns and utilizing problem solving skills to find solutions in case monitoring becomes part of their discharge plan. Monitoring blood glucose is more for the patient than the provider. Monitoring at home should not be used to create anxiety or fear of chronic disease but rather serve as a method for the patient to troubleshoot and evaluate behavior changes.

Reducing risks refers to identifying risks and implementing behaviors to prevent adverse outcomes related to hypoglycemia, hyperglycemia, diabetic ketoacidosis, hyperosmolar hyperglycemic state, retinopathy, nephropathy, neuropathy and cardiovascular complications.[8]

Delivery of diabetes education during hospitalization needs to be given in reasonable amounts to avoid information overload. Survival skills necessary for discharge include addressing how to recognize and treat hypoglycemia. Nursing staff may encourage and offer the opportunity to continue diabetes education outpatient to target more in-depth training in short and long term complications associated with diabetes. The aim for nursing staff is to contribute to a safe discharge.

Problem solving includes the development of a set of strategies by selecting, applying and evaluating the selected strategy for effectiveness. PWD's typically should have a good grasp of the previous 6 behaviors in order to feel confident with problem solving strategies. Hospitalized patients need assistance with survival skills problem solving and shift continued education to outpatient settings. Inpatient diabetes education is an introduction to diabetes education and informing patients of available resources to manage a chronic disease. Oftentimes, inpatient admission is the only exposure to diabetes education. By taking the time to reinforce survival skills and re-attempting to offer the opportunity to establish health coping skills. The patient need reinforcement or refresher training as patient works through barriers.[8]

WHEN

DSME/S is an important component for patients who are frequently hospitalized for treatment of conditions other than diabetes which can aid recovery and safe discharge.[10] A diabetes educator plays an integral part in providing DSME/S. A diabetes educator may be part of an inpatient interdisciplinary team to lead in providing input into patient education, identifying barriers of care, care coordination and transition, nutrition therapy, medication therapy and management, hypoglycemia management and prevention, monitoring glucose control, and professional development.[10] In some cases, a diabetes educator may not be available which is why nursing staff also then becomes a key component and contributor in providing patient education.[10]

Upon completing learning needs assessment, a patient may be quickly identified in early admission process for patient education. By identifying patients early, inpatient team may gather resources to address barriers, offer opportunity for practice and incorporate problem-solving and coping skills.[10] The goal is to prepare the patient or support system to perform survival skills by discharge.[10] Nursing and support staff should not feel overburden to teach all ADCES7 Self-Care Behaviors. Instead the focus should be what does the patient need to safely discharge and transition care to the outpatient setting.

Survival skills which may be provided by nursing staff may include understanding diabetes medication, monitoring blood glucose using glucometer, identifying carbohydrates and treatment of hypoglycemia. The topics can be incorporated and scheduled throughout admission but could also become standard practice in everyday care.

A newly diagnosed patient with diabetes, change in medication or simply providing refresher training on medication can aid compliance, reduce confusion on medication use at discharge and encourage behavior change. Insulin often carries a diabetes stigma on use and administration. Providing a clear message on what insulin is and why it's being injected can guide the conversation on why patients need to use at discharge. Insulin should be described as essential and support staff should aim at removing any negativity associated with a patient needing insulin. Patients often reference insulin use as the worst case scenario and implies the patient is inferior. Insulin may be the quickest method to improve hyperglycemia. Multiple daily injections require frequent monitoring and change in patients routine but it's manageable. Patient education should begin at bedside when insulin is being administered. Nursing staff should identify barriers and attempt to provide ease. For example, a patient may have a fear of needles. Oftentimes, patients have a vision of long needles not realizing needles come in different sizes. Nursing staff may address different sites of injection and discuss different techniques to aid injection such as pinch up methods to reduce discomfort.

Monitoring blood glucose may also become part of the discharge plan. Some health care organizations have resources to provide patients with a sample take home kit which includes a glucometer, lancing device, 10 lancets and 10 testing strips. The benefit of providing a sample kit for take home gives the opportunity to introduce and set up prior to discharge. An education session can also include the teach back method to assess for dexterity and additional barriers.

Nutrition education as part of survival skills can aid patients with menu selections. Primary team may also reach out to the nutrition department by submitting a consult for registered dietitian (RD) visit prior to discharge. Making dietary changes can be challenging for anyone; providers should keep in mind a PWD will need to feel comfortable making changes by using the person-centered approach when developing goals and coping skills. In acute care settings, barriers to optimize glycemic target may include changes in appetite, inconsistency carbohydrate intake, food from outside sources, meal timing and food choices vary from outside environment.[11]

Hypoglycemia can impact patients with or without diabetes which results when blood glucose levels of 70 mg/dL or below. Hypoglycemia can result in cognitive impairment, increased risk for falls, seizures and increased length of stay.[11] Hypoglycemia may be caused by concurrent illness, newly or undiagnosed diabetes, medication error or changes to nutrition.[11] Nursing staff can aid in prevention by providing diabetes education in how to recognize signs or symptoms of hypoglycemia and how to treat without resulting in postprandial hyperglycemia.

WHERE

A health care organization may have a diabetes inpatient service to assist in coordinator care for a PWD but not all do. An interdisciplinary diabetes care team may exist by putting into action appropriate consults during inpatient admission and making best use of provider skills.[12] A pharmacist may assist with resolving medication safety issues, case manager may provide connections to resources and registered dietitian can begin to assess nutritional needs.[12] Nurses need easily accessible resources to complete diabetes education along with simplified charting methods. For example, units may establish a diabetes education teaching toolkit which may include demonstration only insulin pens and approved reputable handouts or booklets. A health care organization may have patient videos accessible inside patients room, mobile device or sent via electronic patient portal. A challenge may be lack of patient education integration into electronic health record (EHR).[13] A health care organization innovative approaches of using electronic tablets with patient education videos.[13] Diabetes educator may be available to provide in-services to units or attend huddle to share brief knowledge and offer encouragement in developing diabetes education skills and techniques. A health care organization needs to establish a desire for change and teamwork approach when offering diabetes education. Access to diabetes educators may be limited but it doesn't mean learning efforts should be canceled. Instead utilize the opportunity to initiate a quality improvement project which can be small scale by one unit and slowly develop across other units. In addition, the desire to engage patients in diabetes education survival skills training can be adopted in routine care.

WHY

Hospital bedside nurses are expected to complete a multitude of tasks and may feel overwhelmed or unprepared to provide "survival skill" training.[14] As a result of limited resources and diabetes education, a patient may leave the hospital without self-care skills and appropriate follow-up care.[14] There is an increased interest in developing effective ways for staff nurses to provide basic DSME/S education and aid in diabetes discharge planning.[14] Nurses agree diabetes education is important but lack of confidence in providing inaccurate information may avoid opportunity with fear patient ask more detailed follow-up questions.[14] Nursing staff also reported lack of time/resources, guidance on expectations, shortened length of stay and managing patient load.[14] But nursing staff spend the most time with patient interaction. Adoption of teaching survival skills into routine care can be acquired by the diabetes team providing continuing education opportunities such as webinars on various diabetes topics to build on knowledge. Improving how we deliver quality patient care becomes easier if we share the opportunities in different patient encounters to encourage behavior change. Nurses shouldn't be the only staff as oftentimes medical assistants (MA) may serve as an additional advocate to providing diabetes education.

SUMMARY

DSME/S is associated with an overall net decrease in overall health care costs and health care organizations should aim at incorporating into routine care.[15,16] Diabetes education provides tools and knowledge to manage diabetes autonomously, improve feeling for treatment and establish shared decision-making between patient and team.[16] Rapid changes in diabetes technology have encouraged adoption of learning more about continuous glucose monitoring (CGM) and insulin pump therapy. Some health care organizations are adapting by developing hospital policies allowing patients to use CGM and insulin pump therapy during inpatient admission which creates more learning opportunities for nursing staff. An adoption of knowledge should be welcomed and not feared. The pandemic of coronavirus disease 2019 (COVID-19) brought on new challenges in how to provide diabetes education to isolated patients.[17] Nursing staff was critically overburdened and seeking assistance with education became limited. Hospitalized COVID-19 patients with hyperglycemia often new to basal/bolus insulin therapy required education on insulin use. Health care organizations and diabetes teams across the world quickly adapted in how to deliver education which included the use of telehealth services. As health care providers we came together to problem solve in order to continue to deliver quality patient care. Providing inpatient diabetes education is essential in developing a discharge plan and has been attributed to reduction in cost in addition to reducing the risk of 30-day readmission.[18] As health care providers and using patient-centered approach, adapting survival skill training into routine care can welcome new hope and encouragement to a PWD. Providing support and taking moments to provide education give a PWD motivation as oftentimes patients feel they are alone managing a chronic disease.

CLINICS CARE POINTS

- DSME is the process of conducting the knowledge and skill necessary for diabetes self-care and DSMS refers the necessary foundation to sustain coping skills and continue behavior to self-manage diabetes.[3]
- An adoption of knowledge should be welcomed and not feared.
- A health care organization needs to establish a desire for change and teamwork approach when offering diabetes education.
- Diabetes management plans should be tailored to the patient's needs and abilities with the aim to slowly push toward the greater goal.

ACKNOWLEDGMENTS

The author would like to acknowledge MD Anderson Cancer Center diabetes team for continued education and practice in providing diabetes education. Our team takes pride in providing quality care using best practices and current research to aid our patients with prime knowledge. Thank you to: Celia Levesque, APP; Seliece Morrow, APP; Sonali Thosani, MD and Victor Lavis, MD.

DISCLOSURES

The author has no relationship with a commercial company that has a direct financial interest in the subject matter or materials discussed in this article or with a company making a competing product.

REFERENCES

1. Korytkowski MT, Muniyappa R, Antinori-Lent K, et al. Management of hyperglycemia in hospitalized adult patients in non-critical care settings: an Endocrine Society clinical practice guideline. J Clin Endocrinol Metabol 2022;107(8):2101–28.
2. Parker ED, Lin J, Mahoney T, et al. Economic costs of diabetes in the US in 2022. Diabetes Care 2024;47(1):26–43.
3. Powers MA, Bardsley J, Cypress M, et al. Diabetes self-management education and support in type 2 diabetes: a joint position statement of the American diabetes association, the American Association of Diabetes Educators, and the Academy of Nutrition and Dietetics. Diabetes Educat 2017;43(1):40–53.
4. Powers MA, Bardsley JK, Cypress M, et al. Diabetes self-management education and support in adults with type 2 diabetes: a consensus report of the American Diabetes Association, the Association of Diabetes Care & Education Specialists, the Academy of Nutrition and Dietetics, the American Academy of Family Physicians, the American Academy of PAs, the American Association of Nurse Practitioners, and the American Pharmacists Association. J Am Pharmaceut Assoc 2020;60(6):e1–18.
5. Kim S, Song Y, Park J, et al. Patients' experiences of diabetes self-management education according to health-literacy levels. Clin Nurs Res 2020;29(5):285–92.
6. Keaveny J. Critical care diabetes education: who, what, when, where, and why. Crit Care Nurs Clin 2013;25(1):123–30.

7. Davis J, Fischl AH, Beck J, et al. 2022 National standards for diabetes self-management education and support. Sci Diabetes Self-Manag Care 2022; 48(1):44–59.
8. Association of Diabetes Care and Education Specialists, Kolb L. An effective model of diabetes care and education: the ADCES7 Self-Care Behaviors™. Sci Diabetes Self-Manag Care 2021;47(1):30–53.
9. Capoccia K, Odegard PS, Letassy N. Medication adherence with diabetes medication: a systematic review of the literature. Diabetes Educat 2016;42(1):34–71.
10. American Association of Diabetes Educators. Role of the diabetes educator in inpatient diabetes management. Diabetes Educat 2018;44(1):57–62.
11. Association of Diabetes Care & Education Specialists. The role of the diabetes care and education specialist in the hospital setting. Sci Diabetes Self Manag Care 2022;48(3):184–91.
12. Hardee SG, Osborne KC, Njuguna N, et al. Interdisciplinary diabetes care: a new model for inpatient diabetes education. Diabetes Spectr 2015;28(4):276–82.
13. Smith KM, Baker KM, Bardsley JK, et al. Redesigning hospital diabetes education: a qualitative evaluation with nursing teams. J Nurs Care Qual 2019;34(2): 151–7.
14. Krall JS, Donihi AC, Hatam M, et al. The Nurse Education and Transition (NEAT) model: educating the hospitalized patient with diabetes. Clin Diabetes and Endocrinol 2016;2:1–6.
15. Whitehouse CR, Haydon-Greatting S, Srivastava SB, et al. Economic impact and health care utilization outcomes of diabetes self-management education and support interventions for persons with diabetes: a systematic review and recommendations for future research. The Science of Diabetes Self-Management and Care 2021;47(6):457–81.
16. Hermanns N, Ehrmann D, Finke-Groene K, et al. Trends in diabetes self-management education: where are we coming from and where are we going? A narrative review. Diabet Med 2020;37(3):436–47.
17. Korytkowski M, Antinori-Lent K, Drincic A, et al. A pragmatic approach to inpatient diabetes management during the COVID-19 pandemic. J Clin Endocrinol Metabol 2020;105(9):3076–87.
18. ElSayed NA, Aleppo G, Aroda VR, et al. 16. Diabetes care in the hospital: standards of care in diabetes—2023. Diabetes Care 2023;46(Supplement_1): S267–78.

Euglycemic Diabetic Ketoacidosis

How Is It Different from Diabetic Ketoacidosis

Hsiao-Hui Ju, DNP, APRN, FNP-BC, CNE

KEYWORDS

- Diabetic ketoacidosis • Euglycemic diabetic ketoacidosis • Diabetes mellitus
- Type 1 • Type 2 • Acidosis • Endocrinology • SGLT-2 inhibitors

KEY POINTS

- Euglycemic DKA can occur when blood glucose levels are less than 200 mg/dL while blood glucose levels exceed 250 mg/dL in DKA.
- The primary pathophysiology mechanism for DKA results from a deficiency of insulin, leading to a rapid onset of marked hyperglycemia-associated symptoms.
- The primary mechanism for euglycemic DKA is a deficiency in carbohydrates, resulting in a reduction of insulin release.
- Any conditions that reduce glucose availability can contribute to euglycemic DKA. Increased glucosuria can lead to a decrease in glucose availability in people taking SGLT-2 inhibitors.
- In euglycemic DKA, there may be a more gradual onset of malaise and vomiting without significant hyperglycemia.

INTRODUCTION, DEFINITIONS, AND BACKGROUND

Diabetic ketoacidosis (DKA) and euglycemic DKA are potentially life-threatening diabetes-related emergencies. It is crucial to distinguish the similarities and differences between the two for accurate diagnosis and evaluation. To prevent serious complications, the healthcare team needs to promptly identify, diagnose, and treat these serious conditions. However, diagnosing euglycemic DKA, especially for people with type 2 diabetes mellitus (T2DM) taking sodium-glucose cotransporter-2 (SGLT-2) inhibitors, may be more challenging due to the absence of substantial hyperglycemia associated with DKA, which is more commonly associated with individuals with type 1 diabetes mellitus (T1DM).[1] As a result, euglycemic DKA may not be considered as a potential diagnosis in individuals with T2DM. Therefore, the pathophysiology,

Department of Undergraduate Studies, The University of Texas at Houston (UTHealth) Cizik School of Nursing, 6901 Bertner Avenue Room #748, Houston, TX 77030, USA
E-mail address: Hsiao-Hui.Ju@uth.tmc.edu

Crit Care Nurs Clin N Am 37 (2025) 157–165
https://doi.org/10.1016/j.cnc.2024.08.004   ccnursing.theclinics.com
0899-5885/25/© 2024 Elsevier Inc. All rights reserved, including those for text and data mining, AI training, and similar technologies.

precipitating factors, clinical presentations, treatment, and evaluations of euglycemic DKA and DKA are reviewed in this article due to the important differences that exist between the two conditions.

DKA is an acute emergency that results from insulin deficiency, leading to severely elevated hyperglycemia and a state of ketoacidosis.[2] Although DKA is more frequently observed in people with T1DM,[3] it can often also be triggered by any metabolic stress or infection in people with T2DM.[2] The substantial hyperglycemia in DKA is typically at levels greater than 250 mg/dL accompanied by metabolic acidosis and ketonemia,[2] accounting for approximately 94% of hospital admissions related to diabetes mellitus.[4] Because of the marked hyperglycemia, patients typically seek immediate medical attention, which results in prompt diagnosis and treatment.

Euglycemic DKA, in contrast, is ketoacidosis with serum glucose levels that are close to normal or in a less severe form of hyperglycemia.[2] Glucose levels can be less than 200[5] or 250 mg/dL[6] in euglycemic DKA (some report a blood glucose upper limit of 250–300 mg/dL, but the blood glucose may be <200 mg/dL).[7,8] At first, euglycemic DKA was documented by Munro and colleagues in 1973 in people with T1DM.[9] However, recently, the use of SGLT-2 inhibitors, a class of medications used in the management of T2DM, has been associated with euglycemic DKA[2] as a number of cases of SGLT-2 inhibitors-treated people with T2DM and euglycemic DKA have been documented.[10] It is estimated that approximately 2.6% to 3.2% of the DKA hospitalizations are patients with euglycemic DKA,[6] but the actual incidence of euglycemic DKA is unknown due to the variation in the serum glucose threshold ranges in the definitions of euglycemic DKA.[2]

PATHOPHYSIOLOGY

Diabetes mellitus (DM) is a chronic metabolic disease due to defects in insulin secretion, action, or both, resulting in hyperglycemia.[11] T1DM is an autoimmune condition where pancreatic β cells are destroyed through T-cell-mediated mechanisms. In contrast, T2DM is characterized by insulin resistance leading to decreased cellular sensitivity to insulin, and can eventually result in the dysfunction of β cells.[11]

Although DKA is more frequently observed in people with T1DM, people with T2DM account for about 25% of the cases.[12] DKA results from a deficiency of insulin, leading to hyperglycemia, glucosuria, dehydration, and electrolyte imbalance.[3] Since serum glucose is unable to enter cells due to an absolute or relative insulin deficiency, the cells release counter-regulatory hormones like glucagon, cortisol, growth hormone, and epinephrine. In response to these counter-regulatory hormones, the liver undergoes glycogenolysis, and proteins and lipids will turn into glucose via gluconeogenesis.[3] As a result, the blood glucose levels continue to rise leading to osmotic diuresis and severe dehydration. In adipocytes, glucose is unable to enter the cells leading to lipolysis with the breakdown of triglycerides and the release of free fatty acids from adipose tissue. In the liver, these free fatty acids undergo beta oxidation, leading to the breakdown of fatty acids into acetyl-CoA, undergoing ketogenesis, and results in the presence of ketone bodies (acetone, acetoacetate, and beta hydroxybutyrate). Consequently, the presence of these highly acidic ketone bodies in the bloodstream ultimately drives the body into metabolic acidosis.[3] In states of stress, including infections, missed insulin doses, physiologic or psychologic stress can trigger DKA in people with T1DM and T2DM.[12]

In euglycemic DKA, there is a deficiency in carbohydrates, which leads to a decrease in serum insulin levels and an increase in counter-regulatory hormones.

Similar to what happens in DKA, an elevated ratio of glucagon to insulin results in the production of ketone bodies from lipolysis leading to ketoacidosis and metabolic acidosis.[2,6] Increased glucosuria by the kidneys or decreased gluconeogenesis by the liver during a state of starvation when glycogen is already depleted also contribute to euglycemic DKA.[6] SGLT-2 inhibitors, a class of medications used in the management of T2DM, have been associated with positive effects on the kidneys and the cardiovascular system, as well as cases of euglycemic DKA.[12,13] They work by increasing renal glucose excretion because they inhibit the reabsorption of glucose and sodium from the proximal renal tubules.[7] Glycosuria as a result of SGLT-2 inhibitors leads to the elimination of a significant amount of glucose from the bloodstream, allowing the body to maintain a relatively normal glucose levels. For people taking SGLT-2 inhibitors, the glycogenolysis and gluconeogenesis are being counteracted by the glucosuria. Since the release of insulin is stimulated by glucose, a reduction in glucose levels leads to a decrease in insulin release. Furthermore, the decrease in extracellular fluid volume from the SGLT-2 inhibitors intensifies the release of counterregulatory hormones.[12] SGLT-2 inhibitors can decrease insulin levels and increase glucagon, which predispose for lipolysis and euglycemic DKA.[1] In the presence of reduced carbohydrate consumption and decreased serum levels of glucose, insulin secretion will be further suppressed.

Pathophysiologic similarities between DKA and euglycemic DKA.

- Both result in the presence of ketone bodies and metabolic acidosis.

Pathophysiology differences include:

- The primary pathophysiology mechanism for DKA results from a deficiency of insulin.
- The primary mechanism for euglycemic DKA is a deficiency in carbohydrates, resulting in a reduction of insulin release. In addition, increased glucosuria can lead to a decrease in glucose availability in people taking SGLT-2 inhibitors.

PRECIPITATING FACTORS

DKA may result from physiologic or psychologic stress or can be the first signs of undiagnosed DM in in some instances.[14] The development of severe hyperglycemia and associated ketoacidosis can be triggered by various risk factors, including infection, missed insulin therapy, and acute serious illnesses such as infarction (myocardial, cerebral), pancreatitis, trauma, pregnancy, thyrotoxicosis, and substance abuse.[13,14] There may be a higher risk for people who take certain medications, such as glucocorticoids, atypical antipsychotics, thiazides, and sympathomimetics, and pentamidine.[13,14] However, infection is considered to be the most common contributing factor in the development of DKA.[13]

Euglycemic DKA can be brought on by any condition that reduces glucose availability, decreases insulin secretion, increases production of counter-regulatory hormones, and increases the ratio of glucagon to insulin.[12] In euglycemic DKA, carbohydrate deprivation and ketosis can result from conditions such as starvation, gastroparesis, and medications such as SGLT-2 inhibitors.[6] With the use of SGLT-2 inhibitors for diabetes treatment, cases of euglycemic DKA have been identified, which led to warnings from the Food and Drug Administration and the European Medicine Agency.[12,15] Additionally, some suggest that euglycemic DKA may occur more frequently in the first 2 months of treatment, even though it might arise at any point after starting SGLT-2 inhibitors.[12] When taking SGLT-2 inhibitors, individuals with a lower body mass index and reduced glycogen stores may be more susceptible to euglycemic

DKA.[6,7,12] Specifically, females were treated for SGLT-2 inhibitor-related ketosis at a higher rate than that of males.[1] Similar to DKA, conditions that causes stress can also trigger euglycemic DKA, such as changes to insulin dose, pancreatitis, infection, surgery, starvation, pregnancy, and substance abuse.[2,6,12]

Precipitating factors similarities between DKA and euglycemic DKA.

- Stress can trigger both DKA and euglycemic DKA.

Precipitating factors differences include:

- Infection is a common contributing factor for DKA.
- Any conditions that reduce glucose availability can contribute to euglycemic DKA.

CLINICAL MANIFESTATIONS AND PHYSICAL EXAMINATION

The clinical manifestations of DKA and euglycemic DKA share many similarities, with a few differences. The onset of DKA can happen quickly and individuals often exhibit symptoms associated with marked hyperglycemia of blood glucose levels greater than 250 mg/dL,[3,13] such as polyuria, polydipsia, and weight loss.[3,13] With inadequate insulin and increasing hyperglycemia, the loss of volume can lead to signs of dehydration, including delayed capillary refill, poor skin turgor, dry mouth, and decreased sweating.[3,13] Anorexia, nausea, vomiting, and abdominal pain are also common.[3,13] If DKA is precipitated by an acute illness, symptoms of infection such as fever, urinary symptoms, abdominal pain, dyspnea, or cough may be present and require a careful assessment.[3] Social history including alcohol consumption and history of substance use should be obtained. While blood pressure can fluctuate, tachycardia and tachypnea are usually noted.[3] Hypotension and tachycardia may be possible, particularly in patients who are experiencing severe dehydration and a serious infection.[13] Kussmaul breathing, characterized by deep and labored breathing, may be observed as a means for the body to compensate for the metabolic acidosis.[6] As a result, a "fruity odor" to the patient's breath, suggesting the presence of acetone, may be noted.[3] Altered mental status such as stupor or coma would indicate severe DKA.[12]

An important distinction for euglycemic DKA is the lack of severe hyperglycemia with blood glucose often less than 200 mg/dL,[7] so patients may not manifest the typical symptoms of polyuria and polydipsia or be mild in intensity.[7] Compared to DKA, euglycemic DKA symptoms may appear more gradually.[7,13] While patients may manifest with malaise, nausea, vomiting, loss of appetite, and signs of dehydration, vomiting is the most common symptom.[15] Their symptoms may also resemble those with DKA and include abdominal pain, dyspnea, Kussmaul breathing, tachycardia, and tachypnea due to the ketoacidosis.[2] People who take SGLT-2 inhibitors may not experience noticeable hyperglycemia, and the use of these medications will further disguise polyuria and polydipsia since these medications works by excreting renal glucose. When euglycemic DKA is compared to DKA, the renal clearance of glucose is about twice as high.[7] Therefore, a detailed history of medications, including adherence or changes to the prescriptions and dosages, should also be obtained.[3] Careful consideration should be given to people with associated risk factors, such as the use of SGLT-2 inhibitors, starvation, pregnancy, alcoholism, and infection.[2] The lack of significant hyperglycemia may also contribute to a delay in the seeking care and in the diagnosis of euglycemic DKA.[7,15]

Clinical manifestations and physical examinations similarities between DKA and euglycemic DKA.

- In both conditions, there are signs of dehydration.
- Due to the metabolic acidosis, Kussmaul breathing, tachycardia, tachypnea can occur in both.

Clinical manifestations and physical examinations differences include:

- In DKA, the rapid onset of the marked hyperglycemia-associated symptoms includes polyuria, polydipsia, and weight loss.
- In euglycemic DKA, there may be a more gradual onset of malaise and vomiting without significant hyperglycemia.

DIAGNOSIS

DKA is characterized by the presence of blood glucose greater than 250 mg/dL, increased anion gap metabolic acidosis (arterial pH less than 7.3, serum bicarbonate less than 18 mEq/L, anion gap >10 mEq/L), and ketonemia or greater than or equal to 2+ urine ketones.[12] Euglycemic DKA involves relative euglycemia (some report a blood glucose upper limit of 250–300 mg/dL, but the blood glucose may be <200 mg/dL[7]), ketonemia or greater than or equal to 2+ urine ketones,[12] and increased anion gap metabolic acidosis (arterial pH less than 7.3, serum bicarbonate less than 18 mEq/L, anion gap >10 mEq/L). Euglycemic DKA was initially documented by Munro and colleagues in 1973,[9,12,15] and subsequently, a more extensive case series was published in 1993.[12,15,16]

There is an approximate 0.65% to 3.3% mortality rate for DKA, with a prevalence of about 4.6 to 8.0 per 1000 patient-years.[7] Depending on the upper cut-off for blood glucose levels, about 2.6% to 7% of patients with DKA were euglycemic.[12,15] The exact incidence of euglycemic DKA is unknown.[12] Without the significant hyperglycemia leading to potential for delayed care and unrecognized diagnosis, euglycemic DKA may be associated with worse outcomes compared to DKA.[7] Therefore, euglycemic DKA should be considered in patients with DM who may have predisposing factors or unexplained high anion gap metabolic acidosis.[2]

If there is a clinical suspicion for DKA or euglycemic DKA, healthcare providers should obtain a careful history with a comprehensive medication list and note if there are any changes to dosages or frequency.[7] Any conditions that may increase a person to metabolic stress should be also identified. Laboratory work-up should be obtained to assess blood glucose, electrolytes, renal function, ketone bodies, complete blood counts, and any other necessary tests based on the specific clinical presentation.[12]

For DKA, blood serum glucose levels are greater than 250 mg/dL. Initially, serum potassium may be normal or elevated due to metabolic acidosis and shifting of intracellular potassium into the plasma, as well as insulin deficiency[3,13] Eventually, hypokalemia may develop due to the total body potassium deficiency.[3] In addition, "pseudohyponatremia" may occur due to the osmosis effect of water being drawn out of cells as a result of hyperglycemia.[13] Thus, sodium may be falsely lowered by 1.6 mEq for every 100 mg/dL increase of blood glucose.[3] For example, to adjust for the pseudohyponatremia in blood glucose level of 600 and serum sodium of 130, the adjusted sodium is 130 + 1.6*5 = 138 mEq/L.

In euglycemic DKA, blood glucose levels are less than 200 to 250 mg/dL[7,13,17] Serum potassium may be normal or low due to potassium depletion.[17] Hyponatremia may occur to a lesser extent compared with DKA.[17] Individuals who are using SGLT2 inhibitors may experience reabsorption of urine ketones instead of their excretion in the urine, which could lead to a false negative result.[12,15] The American College of

Endocrinology recommends using beta-hydroxybutyrate and serum pH to identify euglycemic DKA.[12,15,18] An abnormal serum beta-hydroxybutyrate is greater than 3 mmol/L.[12,15]

In both DKA and euglycemic DKA, acidosis is consistent with a serum pH less than 7.3.[13,17] Bicarbonate is typically less than 18 mEq/L in both,[12,17] but the presence of corrective metabolic alkalosis may be present in people with chronic obstructive pulmonary disease.[13] Three ketone bodies—acetone, acetoacetate, and beta-hydroxybutyrate—are formed during ketoacidosis. The recommended test is beta-hydroxybutyrate, as it is responsible for about 75% of ketones present.[19] The nitroprusside method is not considered the ideal approach because it measures acetoacetate.[15] In both DKA and euglycemic DKA, the presence of ketones contributes to an elevated anion gap (>10 mEq/L).[12,13] Leukocytosis of 10,000 to 15,000 may be seen from dehydration in both.[17] An infectious work-up should be conducted if leukocytosis exceeds 25,000 or bandemia exceeds 10%.[13,17] Renal function tests including blood urea nitrogen and creatinine levels can be elevated in both as a result of dehydration and hypovolemia. Serum magnesium may be low and often needs to be treated in both.[3,6,13] Lastly, phosphate replacement may not improve outcome or duration of DKA in most cases.[3]

The patient's clinical presentation may determine the use of possible imaging studies and diagnostic tests such as electrocardiogram, ultrasound, chest radiograph, and computed tomography.[13] In addition, blood cultures, urinalysis, serum lactate levels, pancreatic or cardiac enzymes, and inflammatory markers may also be obtained in determining the differential diagnosis.[13] In the setting of severe hyperglycemia, hyperosmolar hyperglycemic state may also be considered.

TREATMENT

DKA and euglycemic DKA are treated similarly involving fluid resuscitation, correction of electrolyte imbalances, and infusion of intravenous insulin.[12] Dextrose with insulin is necessary in euglycemic DKA to prevent hypoglycemia that may result from insulin infusion.[7,12] Individuals that developed euglycemic DKA with the use of SGLT-2 inhibitors should carefully assess their diabetes management.[12] A thorough evaluation of the potential risks and benefits of SGLT-2 inhibitors should be made. If the patient is at high risk of recurrence, careful consideration should be taken, and any precipitating factors should be addressed.[12] If the decision was to resume SGLT-2 inhibitors, it is not advisable to restart the treatment immediately right after euglycemic DKA, as this was linked to recurrence or symptomatic ketosis, especially if the insulin dose is not adequate.[7] If there were no additional euglycemic DKA precipitating factors, it is recommended to avoid restarting the medications if the risks of reoccurrences are high.[12]

Initially, intravenous fluids should be started to treat the severe dehydration in both DKA and euglycemic DKA. Normal saline 0.9%, an isotonic solution, may be given for fluid resuscitation for the first 1 to 2 h.[12] After that time, if corrected serum sodium levels are normal or high, use a 0.45% sodium chloride solution.[12] If the corrected sodium levels remain low, normal saline may be continued.[12] Some studies indicated that the use of 0.9% normal saline may result in hyperchloremic non-anion gap metabolic acidosis.[13,15] Furthermore, a crystalloid solution, such as Lactated Ringers, PlasmaLyte, has been found to achieve a sooner resolution of DKA,[20] and may be recommended for use.[13,15]

In addition, basic metabolic panel and serum glucose need to be frequently monitored for electrolyte imbalance, glucose levels, acidosis, and renal function. Due to dilution from the osmotic effect of water being drawn out of cells as a result of hyper-glycemia, serum sodium levels may appear falsely low. Serum sodium may be falsely lowered by 1.6 mEq for every 100 mg/dL increase of blood glucose.[3] For example, to adjust for the pseudohyponatremia in blood glucose level of 600 and serum sodium of 130, the adjusted sodium is 130 + 1.6*5 = 138 mEq/L. In euglycemic DKA, hypona-tremia may occur to a lesser extent and be mild.[17] A different formula recommends using a correction factor of 2.4 mEq/L of for every 100 mg/dL of glucose concentration increase.[13,21] Treat the hyponatremia only if the sodium level remains low after the hyponatremia has been corrected.

Potassium replacement is needed first before starting insulin infusion if serum po-tassium is lesser than 3.5 mEq/L. If the serum potassium level is between 3.5 and 5.5 mEq/L, potassium supplementation should be maintained intravenously to keep the level between 4 and 5 mEq/L.[12,15] If serum potassium is greater than 3.5 mEq/L, an insulin infusion can be initiated.[12] To reduce the risk of hypoglycemia and prevent starving ketosis, dextrose infusion—5% dextrose[15] or 10% dextrose water[7]—also needs to be started.[7] Subcutaneous basal insulin may be initiated when patients are able to tolerate oral food intake and the acidosis resolves to a pH of greater than 7.3 units and serum bicarbonate level greater than 18 mEq/L.[12] To prevent hyper-glycemia, intravenous insulin infusion should be maintained for 1 to 2 h after starting the subcutaneous insulin.[12] Cardiac monitoring and urine output monitoring are necessary during potassium replacement and fluid resuscitation.

PATIENT EDUCATION

Patients with DM should be provided with comprehensive information regarding their treatment plans, including instructions on what to monitor and when to inform their healthcare team. If a patient is receiving insulin treatment, it is crucial to emphasize the necessity of the prescribed insulin usage. Additional important teaching topics include precipitating factors of DKA and euglycemic DKA, the potential signs and symptoms to monitor for each, and the appropriate strategies to manage during pe-riods of illness. If patients begin to not feel well, they should be taught to check their blood glucose closely and consider monitoring their urine for ketones.[7] They should be informed about the precipitating factors, symptoms of euglycemic DKA, and in-structions on when to seek medical attention as euglycemic DKA is possible even in cases where blood glucose levels are near normal or mildly elevated.[7] Individuals with diabetes on SGLT-2 inhibitors should receive instructions on monitoring for the presence of ketones in their urine and blood at the onset of an illness, regardless of their blood glucose levels.[10] Patients should be informed about the potential for euglycemic DKA and be knowledgeable about SGLT-2 inhibitors, the importance of carbohydrate intake, and any findings that would warrant immediate medical attention.[10]

SUMMARY

In conclusion, while DKA and euglycemic DKA share many similarities in their clinical presentations and management, they vary in terms of the serum glucose threshold, pathophysiology, and diagnostic criteria of each condition. The presence of near normal glucose levels in euglycemic DKA differentiates it from the substantial elevated hyperglycemia observed in DKA, which is responsible for the classic symptoms exhibited during its presentation. People with DM, particularly those who have a higher risk of developing euglycemic DKA, should be informed of the potential risk factors, signs and symptoms, and the circumstances under which they should seek medical attention. Lastly, patients should continue to engage in an active discussion with their healthcare team regarding their diabetes medications and treatment plans, taking into account the potential risks and benefits of each option based on their individual health needs and steps to take to prevent any complications.

Unlike DKA, which is characterized by a classic marked hyperglycemia, euglycemic DKA can occur when serum glucose levels are mildly elevated or close to normal. Especially during periods of stress, euglycemic DKA can occur through several pathophysiology mechanisms, including carbohydrate deficit, insulin deficiency, and increased glucagon to insulin ratio.[2] Acute stressors, the use of SGLT-2 inhibitors, starvation or fasting, pregnancy, substance abuse, and surgery have been associated with euglycemic DKA.[2] Delayed treatment of euglycemic DKA may be due to the lack of the noticeable hyperglycemia.[2] Prompt diagnosis and treatment of these potentially life-threatening conditions will be facilitated by an understanding of the similarities and differences between euglycemic DKA and DKA.

CLINICS CARE POINTS

- Euglycemic DKA can occur when blood glucose levels are less than 200 mg/dL while blood glucose levels exceed 250 mg/dL in DKA.
- The primary pathophysiology mechanism for DKA results from a deficiency of insulin, leading to a rapid onset of marked hyperglycemia-associated symptoms.
- The primary mechanism for euglycemic DKA is a deficiency in carbohydrates, resulting in a reduction of insulin release.
- Any conditions that reduce glucose availability can contribute to euglycemic DKA. Increased glucosuria can lead to a decrease in glucose availability in people taking SGLT-2 inhibitors.
- In euglycemic DKA, there may be a more gradual onset of malaise and vomiting without significant hyperglycemia.

DISCLOSURES

The author has nothing to disclose.

REFERENCES

1. Bamgboye AO, Oni IO, Collier A. Predisposing factors for the development of diabetic ketoacidosis with lower than anticipated glucose levels in type 2 diabetes patients on SGLT2-inhibitors: a review. Eur J Clin Pharmacol 2021;77(5):651–7.
2. Nasa P, Chaudhary S, Shrivastava PK, et al. Euglycemic diabetic ketoacidosis: a missed diagnosis. World J Diabetes 2021;12(5):514–23.
3. Lizzo J.M., Goyal A. and Gupta V., Adult Diabetic Ketoacidosis. Updated 2023, In: StatPearls [Internet], 2024, StatPearls Publishing; Treasure Island (FL). Available at: https://www.ncbi.nlm.nih.gov/books/NBK560723/.
4. Khan AA, Ata F, Iqbal P, et al. Clinical and biochemical predictors of intensive care unit admission among patients with diabetic ketoacidosis. World J Diabetes 2023;14(3):271–8.
5. Ogawa W, Sakaguchi K. Euglycemic diabetic ketoacidosis induced by SGLT2 inhibitors: possible mechanism and contributing factors. J Diabetes Investig 2016;7(2):135–8.

6. Plewa M.C., Bryant M. and King-Thiele R., Euglycemic diabetic ketoacidosis, 2023, StatPearls. Treatsure Island (FL): StatPearls. Available at: https://www.ncbi.nlm.nih.gov/books/NBK554570/.
7. Chow E, Clement S, Garg R. Euglycemic diabetic ketoacidosis in the era of SGLT-2 inhibitors. BMJ Open Diabetes Res Care 2023;11(5).
8. Bonora BM, Avogaro A, Fadini GP. Euglycemic ketoacidosis. Curr Diab Rep 2020;20(7):25.
9. Munro JF, Campbell IW, McCuish AC, et al. Euglycaemic diabetic ketoacidosis. Br Med J 1973;2(5866):578–80.
10. Rosenstock J, Ferrannini E. Euglycemic diabetic ketoacidosis: a predictable, detectable, and preventable safety concern with SGLT2 inhibitors. Diabetes Care 2015;38(9):1638–42.
11. Banday MZ, Sameer AS, Nissar S. Pathophysiology of diabetes: an overview. Avicenna J Med Oct-Dec 2020;10(4):174–88.
12. Dagdeviren M, Akkan T, Ertugrul DT. Re-emergence of a forgotten diabetes complication: euglycemic diabetic ketoacidosis. Turk J Emerg Med Jan-Mar 2024;24(1):1–7.
13. Lowie BJ, Bond MC. Diabetic ketoacidosis. Emerg Med Clin North Am 2023; 41(4):677–86.
14. Ghimire P. and Dhamoon A.S., Ketoacidosis, 2024, StatPearls. Treasure Island (FL): StatPearls. Available at: https://www.ncbi.nlm.nih.gov/books/NBK534848/.
15. Long B, Lentz S, Koyfman A, et al. Euglycemic diabetic ketoacidosis: etiologies, evaluation, and management. Am J Emerg Med 2021;44:157–60.
16. Jenkins D, Close CF, Krentz AJ, et al. Euglycaemic diabetic ketoacidosis: does it exist? Acta Diabetol 1993;30(4):251–3.
17. Jarvis PRE. Euglycemic diabetic ketoacidosis: a potential pitfall for the emergency physician. Clin Exp Emerg Med 2023;10(1):110–3.
18. Handelsman Y, Henry RR, Bloomgarden ZT, et al. American association of clinical endocrinologists and American College of Endocrinology position statement on the association of sglt-2 inhibitors and diabetic ketoacidosis. Endocr Pract 2016;22(6): 753–62.
19. EL-Mohandes N., Yee G., Bhutta B.S., et al., Pediatric diabetic ketoacidosis, 2024, StatPearls, StatPearls Publishing; Treasure Island (FL). Available at: https://www.ncbi.nlm.nih.gov/books/NBK470282/.
20. Self WH, Evans CS, Jenkins CA, et al. Clinical effects of balanced crystalloids vs saline in adults with diabetic ketoacidosis: a subgroup analysis of cluster randomized clinical trials. JAMA Netw Open 2020;3(11):e2024596.
21. Hillier TA, Abbott RD, Barrett EJ. Hyponatremia: evaluating the correction factor for hyperglycemia. Am J Med 1999;106(4):399–403.

Moving?

Make sure your subscription moves with you!

To notify us of your new address, find your **Clinics Account Number** (located on your mailing label above your name), and contact customer service at:

Email: journalscustomerservice-usa@elsevier.com

800-654-2452 (subscribers in the U.S. & Canada)
314-447-8871 (subscribers outside of the U.S. & Canada)

Fax number: 314-447-8029

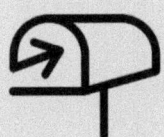

Elsevier Health Sciences Division
Subscription Customer Service
3251 Riverport Lane
Maryland Heights, MO 63043

*To ensure uninterrupted delivery of your subscription, please notify us at least 4 weeks in advance of move.

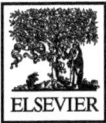

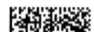